Soft Tissue Pathology

Editor

GREGORY W. CHARVILLE

SURGICAL PATHOLOGY CLINICS

www.surgpath.theclinics.com

Consulting Editor
JASON L. HORNICK

March 2024 • Volume 17 • Number 1

ELSEVIER

1600 John F. Kennedy Boulevard • Suite 1800 • Philadelphia, Pennsylvania, 19103-2899

http://www.theclinics.com

SURGICAL PATHOLOGY CLINICS Volume 17, Number 1
March 2024 ISSN 1875-9181, ISBN-13: 978-0-443-18388-1

Editor: Taylor Hayes
Developmental Editor: Saswoti Nath

Surgical Pathology Clinics (ISSN 1875-9181) is published quarterly by Elsevier Inc., 360 Park Avenue South, New York, NY 10010. Months of issue are March, June, September, and December. Business and Editorial Office: Elsevier Inc., 1600 John F. Kennedy Blvd., Ste. 1800, Philadelphia, PA 19103-2899. Accounting and Circulation Offices: Elsevier Inc., 3251 Riverport Lane, Maryland Heights, MO 63043. Periodicals postage paid at New York, NY and at additional mailing offices. Subscription prices are $253.00 per year (US individuals), $100.00 per year (US students/residents), $294.00 per year (Canadian individuals), $307.00 per year (foreign individuals), and $120.00 per year (international students/residents), $100.00 per year (Canadian students/residents). For institutional access pricing please contact Customer Service via the contact information below. Foreign air speed delivery is included in all *Clinics*' subscription prices. All prices are subject to change without notice. **POSTMASTER:** Send address changes to *Surgical Pathology Clinics*, Elsevier, 3251 Riverport Lane, Maryland Heights, MO 63043. **Customer Service: 1-800-654-2452 (US). From outside the United States, call 1-314-447-8871. Fax: 1-314-447-8029. E-mail:** JournalsCustomerServiceusa@elsevier. com **(for print support)** and JournalsOnlineSupport-usa@elsevier.com **(for online support)**.

Reprints. For copies of 100 or more, of articles in this publication, please contact the Commercial Reprints Department, Elsevier Inc., 360 Park Avenue South, New York, NY 10010-1710. Tel. 212-633-3874; Fax: 212-633-3820; E-mail: reprints@elsevier.com.

Surgical Pathology Clinics of North America is covered in *MEDLINE/PubMed (Index Medicus)*.

Contributors

CONSULTING EDITOR

JASON L. HORNICK, MD, PhD
Director of Surgical Pathology and
Immunohistochemistry, Brigham and Women's
Hospital, Professor of Pathology, Harvard
Medical School, Boston, Massachusetts, USA

EDITOR

GREGORY W. CHARVILLE, MD, PhD
Assistant Professor, Department of Pathology,
Stanford University School of Medicine,
Stanford, California, USA

AUTHORS

SCOTT C. BRESLER, MD, PhD
Assistant Professor, Departments of Pathology
and Dermatology, University of Michigan,
Ann Arbor, Michigan, USA

JULIA A. BRIDGE, MD
Department of Pathology and Microbiology,
University of Nebraska Medical Center,
Omaha, Nebraska, USA; Division of Molecular
Pathology, ProPath, Dallas, Texas, USA

GREGORY W. CHARVILLE, MD, PhD
Assistant Professor, Department of Pathology,
Stanford University School of Medicine,
Stanford, California, USA

ELEANOR Y. CHEN, MD, PhD
Associate Professor, Department of
Laboratory Medicine and Pathology, University
of Washington, Seattle, Washington, USA

JEFFREY M. CLOUTIER, MD, PhD
Assistant Professor of Pathology, Department
of Pathology and Laboratory Medicine,
Dartmouth Hitchcock Medical Center,
Lebanon, New Hampshire, USA; Dartmouth
Geisel School of Medicine, Hanover, New
Hampshire, USA

JOSEPHINE K. DERMAWAN, MD, PhD
Associate Staff, Robert J. Tomsich Pathology
and Laboratory Medicine Institute, Cleveland
Clinic, Cleveland, Ohio, USA

**MARÍA PURIFICACIÓN DOMÍNGUEZ
FRANJO, MD, PhD**
Medical Director, Pathology Department,
Hospital Ruber Internacional, Madrid, Spain

ANDREW L. FOLPE, MD
Pathologist, Department of Pathology and
Laboratory Medicine, Mayo Clinic, Rochester,
Minnesota, USA

PHOEBE M. HAMMER, MD
Resident, Department of Pathology, Stanford
University School of Medicine, Stanford,
California, USA

ANDREW HORVAI, MD, PhD
Clinical Professor, Pathology, University of
California, San Francisco, San Francisco,
California, USA

ISABELLE HOSTEIN, PhD
Department of Biopathology, Institut Bergonié,
Comprehensive Cancer Center, Bordeaux,
France

ERICA Y. KAO, MD
Pathologist, Department of Pathology, Brooke
Army Medical Center, San Antonio, Texas,
USA

DARCY A. KERR, MD
Associate Professor of Pathology, Department
of Pathology and Laboratory Medicine,
Dartmouth Hitchcock Medical Center,
Lebanon, New Hampshire, USA; Dartmouth
Geisel School of Medicine, Hanover, New
Hampshire, USA

WILLIAM B. LASKIN, MD
Professor, Department of Pathology, Yale
School of Medicine, New Haven, Connecticut,
USA

KONSTANTINOS LINOS, MD
Pathologist, Department of Pathology and
Laboratory Medicine, Memorial Sloan
Kettering Cancer Center, New York, New York,
USA

ANTONIO LLOMBART-BOSCH, MD, PhD
Professor, Pathology Department, University of
Valencia, Spain and Cancer CIBER
(CIBERONC), Madrid, Spain

ISIDRO MACHADO, MD, PhD
Pathology Department, Instituto Valenciano de
Oncología, Patologika Laboratory, Hospital
Quiron-Salud, Pathology Department,
University of Valencia, Valencia, Spain

NAOHIRO MAKISE, MD, PhD
Division of Surgical Pathology, Chiba Cancer
Center, Chiba, Japan

JEANNE M. MEIS, MD
Professor, Department of Pathology and
Laboratory Medicine, The University of Texas
MD Anderson Cancer Center, Houston, Texas,
USA

MICHAEL MICHAL, MD, PhD
Associate Professor, Department of Pathology,
Charles University, Faculty of Medicine in
Plzen, Bioptical Laboratory, Ltd, Plzen, Czech
Republic

SAMUEL NAVARRO, MD, PhD
Pathology Department, University of Valencia,
Spain and Cancer CIBER (CIBERONC),
Madrid, Spain

RAJIV M. PATEL, MD
Professor, Departments of Pathology and
Dermatology, University of Michigan, Ann
Arbor, Michigan, USA; Cutaneous Pathology,
WCP Laboratories, Inc, Maryland Heights,
Missouri, USA

RAUL PERRET, MD, MSc
Department of Biopathology, Institut Bergonié,
Comprehensive Cancer Center, Bordeaux,
France

AMIR QORBANI, MD
Assistant Clinical Professor, Pathology,
University of California, San Francisco, San
Francisco, California,
USA

JASMINE S. SALEH, MD, MPH
Dermatopathology Fellow, Departments of
Pathology and Dermatology, University of
Michigan, Ann Arbor, Michigan, USA

SERENA Y. TAN, MD
Assistant Professor, Department of Pathology,
Stanford University School of Medicine,
Stanford, California, USA

LAURA M. WARMKE, MD
Assistant Professor, Department of Pathology
and Laboratory Medicine, Indiana University,
Indianapolis, Indiana, USA

CARLI P. WHITTINGTON, MD
Dermatopathology Fellow, Departments of
Pathology and Dermatology, University of
Michigan, Ann Arbor, Michigan, USA

HAO WU, MD, PhD
Assistant Professor, Department of Pathology,
Yale School of Medicine, New Haven,
Connecticut, USA

AKIHIKO YOSHIDA, MD, PhD
Assistant Professor, Department of Diagnostic
Pathology, National Cancer Center Hospital,
Tokyo, Japan

WENDONG YU, MD, PhD
Associate Professor, Department of Pathology
and Laboratory Medicine, The University of
Texas MD Anderson Cancer Center, Houston,
Texas, USA

Contents

> Superficial CD34-positive fibroblastic tumor is a mesenchymal neoplasm of "intermediate malignancy" recently included in the fifth edition of the World Health Organization classification of soft tissue and bone tumors. In this review, we summarize the current knowledge on this rare entity with a special focus on its clinicopathological features, morphologic spectrum, and differential diagnosis. We also provide data regarding recent discoveries on its molecular profile and discuss its prognosis and management.

> GLI1-altered mesenchymal tumors comprise an emerging group of neoplasms characterized by fusions or amplifications involving *GLI1*, a gene that encodes a key regulator of the Hedgehog signaling pathway. In recent years, tumors with GLI1 alterations have been reported across a variety of anatomic sites and a broad age range. Although these tumors can exhibit a wide morphologic spectrum and a variable immunophenotype, they frequently present with monomorphic ovoid cells arranged in distinctive nests with a rich, arborizing vascular network. Recent evidence indicates that they have the potential to metastasize, which suggests that they may be best considered a sarcoma.

> Myxoid pleomorphic liposarcoma (MPLPS) shows a strong predilection for the mediastinum and can affect a wide age range. Clinically, MPLPS exhibits aggressive behavior and demonstrates a worse overall and progression-free survival than myxoid/round cell liposarcoma (MRLPS) and pleomorphic liposarcoma (PLPS). Histologically, MPLPS is characterized by hybrid morphologic features of MRLPS and PLPS, including myxoid stroma, chicken wire-like vasculature, univacuolated and multivacuolated lipoblasts, and high-grade pleomorphic sarcomatous components. In terms of molecular features, MPLPS is distinct from other lipomatous tumors as it harbors genome-wide loss of heterozygosity.

> The wide application of increasingly advanced molecular studies in routine clinical practice has allowed a detailed, albeit still incomplete, genetic subclassification of undifferentiated round cell sarcomas. The WHO classification continues to include provisional molecular entities, whose clinicopathologic features are in the early stages of evolution. This review focuses on the clinicopathologic, molecular, and prognostic features of undifferentiated round cell sarcomas with *EWSR1/FUS::N-FATC2* or *EWSR1::PATZ1* fusions. Classic histopathologic findings, uncommon variations, and diagnostic pitfalls are addressed, along with the utility of recently developed immunohistochemical and molecular markers.

Xanthogranulomatous epithelial tumor is a recently described soft tissue tumor characterized by subcutaneous location, partial encapsulation, a xanthogranulomatous inflammatory cell infiltrate, and keratin-positive mononuclear cells. It shares some morphologic features with keratin-positive, giant cell-rich soft tissue tumors. Both have recently been shown to harbor HMGA2::NCOR2 fusions. The relationship between these tumors and their differential diagnosis with other osteoclast-containing soft tissue tumors is discussed.

Inflammatory rhabdomyoblastic tumor is a recently introduced name for neoplasms currently included in the World Health Organization classification of soft tissue tumors under the rubric inflammatory leiomyosarcoma. Inflammatory rhabdomyoblastic tumor is an excellent example of how surgical pathologists working in conjunction with tumor biologists can greatly improve tumor classification to the benefit of patients. Over the last 28 years, understanding of this entity has undergone a fascinating evolution. This review serves as a summary of the latest findings in inflammatory rhabdomyoblastic tumor research and a diagnostic manual for the practicing surgical pathologist.

Calcified chondroid mesenchymal neoplasms (CCMN) represent a morphologic spectrum of related tumors. Historically, chondroid matrix or chondroblastoma-like features have been described in soft tissue chondroma, tenosynovial giant cell tumors (especially of the temporomandibular joint (TMJ) region), and in a subset of tophaceous pseudogout. Recently, these tumors have been found to share FN1-receptor tyrosine kinase (RTK) fusions. This review discusses the clinical, morphologic, immunohistochemical, and molecular genetic features of CCMN. The distinction from morphologic mimics is also discussed.

MIFS is a low-grade fibroblastic sarcoma that predilects to superficial distal extremity soft tissue. It is composed of plump spindled and epithelioid cells, inflammatory infiltrates, and mucin deposits in a fibrosclerotic stroma. Large epithelioid cells harboring bizarre nuclei and virocyte-like macronucleoli and pleomorphic pseudolipoblasts are characteristic. While conventional MIFS has locally recurrent potential but minimal metastatic risk, tumors with high-grade histologic features have a greater risk for recurrence and metastasis. Wide local excision is the recommended treatment.

Atypical spindle cell/pleomorphic lipomatous tumor (ASCPLT) is a rare soft tissue neoplasm, commonly arising in the subcutis (more common than deep soft tissue) of limbs and limb girdles during mid-adulthood. ASCPLT is histologically a lipogenic neoplasm with ill-defined margins composed of a variable amount of spindle to pleomorphic/multinucleated cells within a fibromyxoid stroma. ASCPLTs lack *MDM2* amplification, but a large subset show *RB1* deletion and variable expression of CD34. Though initially thought to be the malignant form of spindle cell lipoma, ASCPLTs are benign with local recurrences ($\sim$10-15%) and no well-documented dedifferentiation or metastasis.

Perivascular epithelioid cell tumors (PEComas) are a heterogenous group of mesenchymal neoplasms with a mixed myomelanocytic immunophenotype. PEComa-family tumors include angiomyolipoma, lymphangioleiomyomatosis, and a large category of rare neoplasms throughout the body that are now classified under the umbrella term "PEComa." This review focuses on recent advances in the clinicopathological and molecular features of PEComas, with an emphasis on PEComas that originate in soft tissue.

Sclerosing epithelioid fibrosarcoma (SEF) is a distinctive sarcoma that may arise in nearly any soft tissue site or bone. While there has been past controversy as to whether it is related to low-grade fibromyxoid sarcoma (LGFMS), it has been shown to behave far more aggressively than LGFMS. SEF has a propensity to metastasize to the lungs and bone and arise within the abdominal cavity. Histologically, it is characterized by uniform nuclei embedded in a densely collagenous stroma simulating osteoid. By immunohistochemistry, it is often strongly positive for MUC4. The majority (75%) have EWSR1 gene rearrangement, most commonly with CREB3L1 as a fusion partner, although a variety of FUS/EWSR1 and CREB3L1/CREB3L2/CREB3L3 fusions have been described in addition to others. SEF is currently recalcitrant to nearly all chemotherapy and radiation therapy.

CIC-rearranged sarcoma is a rare type of small round cell sarcoma. The tumors often affect the deep soft tissues of patients in a wide age range. They are highly aggressive, respond poorly to chemotherapy, and have a worse outcome than Ewing sarcoma. *CIC*-rearranged sarcoma has characteristic and recognizable histology, including lobulated growth, focal myxoid changes, round to epithelioid cells, and minimal variation of nuclear size and shape. Nuclear ETV4 and WT1 expression are useful immunohistochemical findings. *CIC* fusion can be demonstrated using various methods; however, even next-generation sequencing suffers from imperfect sensitivity, especially for *CIC::DUX4*.

Pleomorphic dermal sarcoma (PDS) is a rare cutaneous/subcutaneous neoplasm of purported mesenchymal differentiation that exists along a clinicopathologic spectrum with atypical fibroxanthoma (AFX). While PDS and AFX share histopathologic and immunohistochemical features, PDS exhibits deeper tissue invasion and has a higher rate of metastasis and local recurrence than AFX. Given its aggressive clinical course, early recognition and clinical management of PDS are essential for optimizing patient outcomes. This review aims to provide a brief overview of the clinicopathologic and molecular features, prognosis, and treatment of PDS.

SURGICAL PATHOLOGY CLINICS

SERIES OF RELATED INTEREST

Clinics in Laboratory Medicine
http://www.labmed.theclinics.com/
Medical Clinics
https://www.medical.theclinics.com/

THE CLINICS ARE AVAILABLE ONLINE!
Access your subscription at:
www.theclinics.com

Preface
Frontiers in Soft Tissue Tumor Pathology

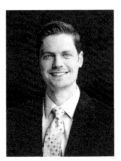

Gregory W. Charville, MD, PhD
Editor

Soft tissue pathology encompasses an exceptionally diverse array of histologically, clinically, and molecularly distinctive neoplasms. With careful morphologic studies now increasingly buttressed by high-throughput approaches for molecular analysis, the list of soft tissue tumor entities seemingly grows by the day, even as our understanding of existing entities continues to evolve. This rapid growth of knowledge, daunting as it may seem, offers the opportunity for pathologists to have an increasingly impactful role in driving appropriate treatment of even the rarest of tumors.

Effectively implementing this new knowledge requires that we take stock of what has recently been learned and what remains to be understood. The goal of this issue is to do just that, by offering expert soft tissue pathologists—those whose work has fueled our understanding of these emerging and evolving entities—a venue to share the current state of their own knowledge, and how that knowledge manifests in their daily practice.

The individual articles that comprise this issue reflect the diversity and breadth of soft tissue tumors, including those with lipomatous, fibroblastic, and myogenic differentiation, along with those that are histologically undifferentiated. There are some articles dedicated to our newly evolved understanding of well-established entities, and others that focus on entirely novel tumor types. Several articles tell the fascinating story of discovery, of initially disconnected observations and insights that ultimately converged into a well-defined and recognizable diagnostic standard. Although molecular pathology is a theme that features prominently in each of the articles, the authors collectively highlight the primacy of histomorphology both in the original discovery of these entities and in the routine diagnostic approach to them.

Together, this collection of articles is intended to serve not only as a practical guide for physicians and scientists who are navigating the complexities of these emerging and evolving diagnostic entities, but also as a foundation for future studies.

Gregory W. Charville, MD, PhD
Department of Pathology
Stanford University School of Medicine
300 Pasteur Drive, Lane 235
Stanford, CA 94305-5324, USA

E-mail address:
gwc@stanford.edu

https://doi.org/10.1016/j.path.2023.07.005
1875-9181/24/© 2023 Published by Elsevier Inc.

surgpath.theclinics.com

Superficial CD34-Positive Fibroblastic Tumor

Raul Perret, MD, MSc*, Isabelle Hostein, PhD

KEYWORDS

• Superficial CD34-Positive fibroblastic tumor • *PRDM10* • Sarcoma

---

Key points

- Superficial CD34-positive fibroblastic tumor is a recently described lesion predominantly affecting the superficial soft tissues of the limbs of young adults (20–40 years old).
- Prototypical cases are well-circumscribed and composed of sheets and fascicles of spindle to epithelioid cells with pleomorphic nuclei and very low mitotic activity; tumor necrosis is exceptional.
- A variable abundance of granular cell change, myxoid stromal changes, hemosiderin deposits, ectatic blood vessels with damaged walls, lipidized tumor cells, and metaplastic bone can be seen.
- By definition, tumors are diffusely and strongly positive for CD34 and ~70% focally express pan-keratin (AE1-AE3). *PRDM10* gene rearrangements are detected in a variable proportion of cases.
- The prognosis of patients with this tumor is excellent, with local recurrences reported in ~9% of cases and no disease-associated deaths. Metastatic spread to regional lymph nodes has been anecdotally reported.
- The recommended treatment is complete surgical excision with negative margins.

ABSTRACT

Superficial CD34-positive fibroblastic tumor is a mesenchymal neoplasm of "intermediate malignancy" recently included in the fifth edition of the World Health Organization classification of soft tissue and bone tumors. In this review, we summarize the current knowledge on this rare entity with a special focus on its clinicopathological features, morphologic spectrum, and differential diagnosis. We also provide data regarding recent discoveries on its molecular profile and discuss its prognosis and management.

INTRODUCTION

In 2014, Carter and colleagues described for the first time a peculiar mesenchymal neoplasm originating in the superficial somatic soft tissues and showing striking nuclear pleomorphism, a very low mitotic activity, consistent diffuse CD34 expression, and frequent focal cytokeratin expression.[1] In their seminal article, the authors observed that these tumors showed predominantly an indolent clinical course with no disease-associated deaths and only a single case developing metastatic dissemination to a regional lymph node, despite most cases being originally diagnosed as sarcomas. To reflect the distinctive clinicopathological and immunohistochemical features of this neoplasm, the term "Superficial CD34-positive fibroblastic tumor" (CD34FT) was proposed.

After almost 10 years since the original description, more than 150 additional cases of CD34FT have been described in the English literature,[1–10] allowing the confirmation and evolution of the

---

Department of Biopathology, Institut Bergonié, Comprehensive Cancer Center, Bordeaux F-33000, France
* Corresponding author.
E-mail address: r.perret@bordeaux.unicancer.fr
Twitter: @kells108 (R.P.)

Surgical Pathology 17 (2024) 1–12
https://doi.org/10.1016/j.path.2023.06.001
1875-9181/24/© 2023 Elsevier Inc. All rights reserved.

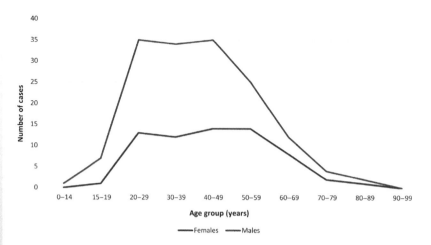

Fig. 1. Superficial CD34-positive fibroblastic tumor: incidence by age and gender (n = 155).

original observations made by Carter and colleagues. In particular, the widespread application of molecular biology has allowed us to more precisely dissect the genetic foundations of CD34FT and identify, among others, the presence of recurrent translocations involving the *PRDM10* gene.

This review summarizes the current knowledge on CD34FT, with an emphasis on its morphologic spectrum, differential diagnosis and molecular underpinnings. The correct identification of CD34FT is of major clinical significance to avoid overtreatment and is readily feasible with careful morphologic assessment and the use of a limited panel of widely available immunohistochemical markers.

CLINICAL FINDINGS

Most cases of CD34FT occur in young adults between their 20s and 40s, but the age range is wide; notably, the pediatric population seems to be rarely affected (**Fig. 1**). There is a male predilection (male-to-female ratio = 1.38:1). Most lesions arise in the lower extremities, the thigh being the most frequent location overall; other sites include the trunk, upper limbs, and head and neck. The viscera and body cavities do not seem to be affected. The most common patient complaint is that of a mass, frequently known for a long period before consultation (months to years). In rare cases, tumors can be painful.[2,6,11]

MACROSCOPIC FEATURES

Most cases present as relatively well-circumscribed superficial (cutaneous/subcutaneous) masses that are generally ≤50 mm in the largest dimension (**Fig. 2**). Occasional cases can be large (up to 100 mm) or bulge into the deep fascia. Furthermore, rare deep (intramuscular) examples have been documented.[2] In general, CD34FT has a homogeneous tan/beige fleshy cut surface (**Fig. 3**), but variable amounts of hemorrhage, myxoid change and cystic degeneration can be seen.

MICROSCOPIC FEATURES

Classic examples of CD34FT (**Fig. 4**) are centered on the dermis or hypodermis and show a nodular or lobulated silhouette which can either be sharply

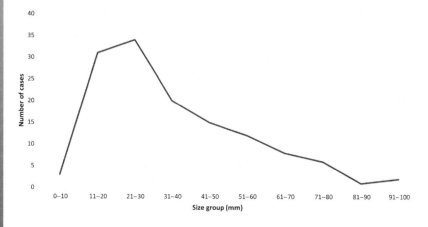

Fig. 2. Superficial CD34-positive fibroblastic tumor: distribution of cases related to tumor size (n = 132).

Fig. 3. Gross findings of a typical case of superficial CD34-positive fibroblastic tumor, scale bar 1 cm. (*Courtesy of* Dr Noelle Weingertner, Strasbourg, France).

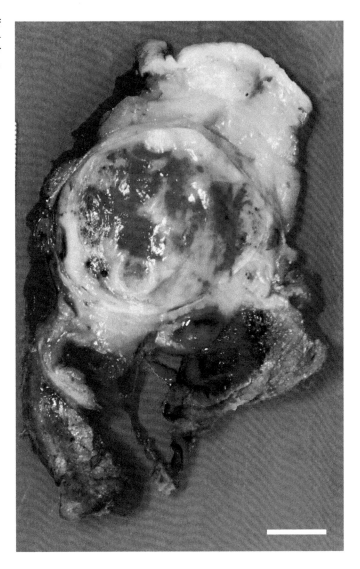

circumscribed from the surrounding stroma (sometimes showing a cleft artifact) or show more irregular (jagged) borders. On low power, lesions have a myoid appearance ("pink tumors") owing to the abundance of eosinophilic cytoplasm of the neoplastic cells. In addition, "satellite" lymphoid aggregates can be frequently appreciated. On higher power, tumors are typically composed of densely cellular sheets and fascicles of spindle to epithelioid cells with well-defined cell borders and abundant eosinophilic cytoplasm, which may have a variable "glassy" or granular appearance. Tumor cell nuclei typically range from moderate to markedly pleomorphic, with heterogeneous chromatin and variably conspicuous nucleoli. Intranuclear pseudoinclusions are frequent, and some cases may present "virocyte-like cells." Importantly, despite the alarming nuclear pleomorphism, necrosis is very rare (**Box 1**), and mitotic activity is typically extremely low, with the vast majority of cases showing less than 1 mitotic figure per mm^2 (see **Box 1**). Interestingly, exceptional cases can show a higher mitotic activity (>1 per mm^2) and atypical mitotic figures, but these findings do not seem to have prognostic significance.[8] Additional variable features include a mixed inflammatory infiltrate, myxoid stromal changes, hemosiderin deposits (which may be massive), ectatic blood vessels with damaged walls, lipidized tumor cells and metaplastic bone.

Notably, several of the histologic findings described above can be widespread throughout the tumor, which can be grouped into morphologic variants of CD34FT.

- Granular cell: while many examples of CD34FT show limited areas of granular cell change, in some cases, this finding can be

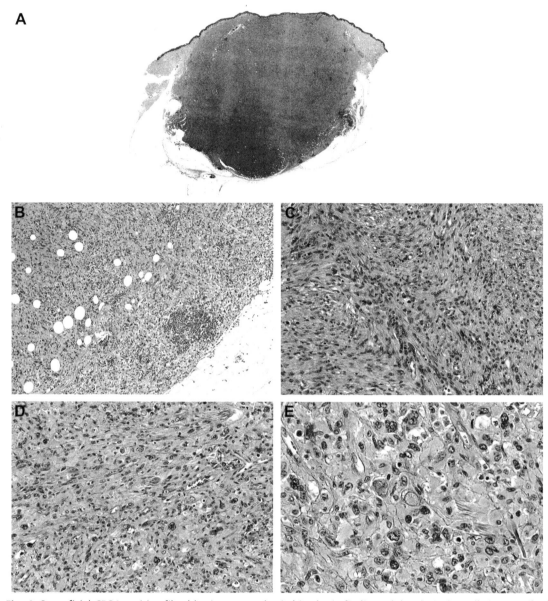

Fig. 4. Superficial CD34-positive fibroblastic tumor: classic histologic findings. (*A*) Relatively well-circumscribed dermo-hypodermic tumor (note the pink color). (*B*) Peripheral lymphoid aggregates. (*C*) and (*D*) fascicles and sheets of spindle to epithelioid cells with pleomorphic nuclei. (*E*) Abundant eosinophilic "glassy" cytoplasm and nuclear pseudoinclusions.

extensive (**Fig. 5**). Importantly, focal areas of classic CD34FT generally can still be identified.

- Lipidized: typically shows tumor cells with abundant, clear, multivacuolated cytoplasm, which may closely mimic lipoblasts (see **Fig. 5**). Aggregates of foamy macrophages are also frequently present.
- Pleomorphic hyalinizing angiectatic tumor (PHAT)-like: this variant shows a variable

abundance of ectatic blood vessels with damaged walls (fibrinous amorphous material deposits) sometimes associated with organizing thrombi (**Fig. 6**). In addition, intracellular and extracellular hemosiderin deposits are frequently present (and can be massive).

- Myxoid: this variant is characterized by a prominent myxoid matrix (**Fig. 7**).
- Spindle cell: in this variant, spindle tumor cells predominate, and nuclear pleomorphism is

Box 1
Summary of clinicopathological features of Superficial CD34-positive fibroblastic tumors reported in the English literature

Number of total cases[a]

  n = 164

Gender (n = 155)

  Female, n = 65

  Male, n = 90

Age (n = 155)

  median 40 y (range: 14–85)

Location (n = 152)

  Thigh, n = 60

  Trunk, n = 22

  Leg, n = 21

  Buttock, n = 10

  Arm, n = 10

  Ankle, n = 5

  Foot, n = 5

  Knee, n = 4

  Forearm, n = 4

  Groin, n = 3

  Neck, n = 3

  Hip, n = 2

  Popliteal fossa, n = 1

  Perineum, n = 1

  Breast, n = 1

Size (mm, n = 132)

  median 30 (range 10–100)

Mitotic activity (per mm², n = 116)

  mean 0.09 mitoses (range 0–3.6)

Necrosis (present/total cases, %)

  1/150; 0.6%

Local recurrence (present/total cases, %)

  9/102; 8.8%

Metastasis (present/total cases, %)

  2/101; 1.9%

Follow-up (months, n = 99)

  median 21 (range 1–231)

[a]Data of all cases was not available for every variable assessed.
References: Carter et al.[1]; Perret et al.[2]; Batur et al.[3]; Puls et al.[4,5]; Lao et al.[6]; Hendry et al.[7]; Anderson et al.[8]; Ding et al.[9]; Zhao et al.[10]; Sugita et al.[13].

generally milder than in classical cases (see **Fig. 7**). Associated myxoid stromal changes are not uncommon.

IMMUNOHISTOCHEMISTRY

By definition, CD34FT is diffusely and strongly positive with CD34 (**Fig. 8**). Around ∼75% of cases are positive with pan-keratin (AE1/AE3) and ∼30 to 50% with desmin.[2,8] Importantly, pan-keratin and desmin are typically focal or multifocal, highlighting tumor cells with dendritic morphology. Most cases express SynCAM3 (*CADM3*), which was initially thought to be exclusive to cases with fusions involving the *PRDM10* gene.[12] However, additional studies have revealed that SynCAM3 positivity is seen in both fusion-positive and -negative cases.[2] Other frequently positive but nonspecific markers include WT1,[8] PRDM10[4] and cyclin D1.[13] Cases showing expression for MDM2 have been reported, but there is no gene amplification.[2] INI-1 (*SMARCB1*) nuclear expression is retained in all cases. The following markers are negative: S100, SOX10, CD31, ERG, ALK, and h-Caldesmon. A detailed list of antibodies tested in CD34FT is shown in **Table 1**.

MOLECULAR FEATURES

The application of molecular biology-based techniques has evidenced that CD34FT shows recurrent rearrangements of the *PRDM10* gene in 37% to 77% of cases (**Fig. 9**).[2,5,8,10] The wide range of positivity is most likely related to the sensitivity of the technique used to detect *PRDM10* rearrangements in FFPE material.[5] In general, *PRDM10* fuses to *MED12* (the most common partner) or *CITED2*, resulting in *MED12/CITED2::PRDM10* gene fusions.[2,5] Isolated cases showing fusions with *RAB30* and *ARHGAP32* have also been reported, and notably, in these examples, *PRDM10* was located at the 5′ end of the fusion gene (ie, *PRDM10::RAB30/ARHGAP32*).[2] A list of fusions reported in CD34FT is presented in **Table 2**.

The PRDM10 protein is a zinc finger transcriptional regulator which modulates gene expression by binding to specific DNA sequences through its zinc finger domain. In vitro studies have demonstrated that *PRDM10* fusions result in a putative chimeric protein that induces the dysregulation of numerous genes, including marked upregulation of *CADM3* (which encodes the SynCAM3 protein).[12] As previously discussed, the latter can be exploited for diagnostic purposes (see immunohistochemistry section).

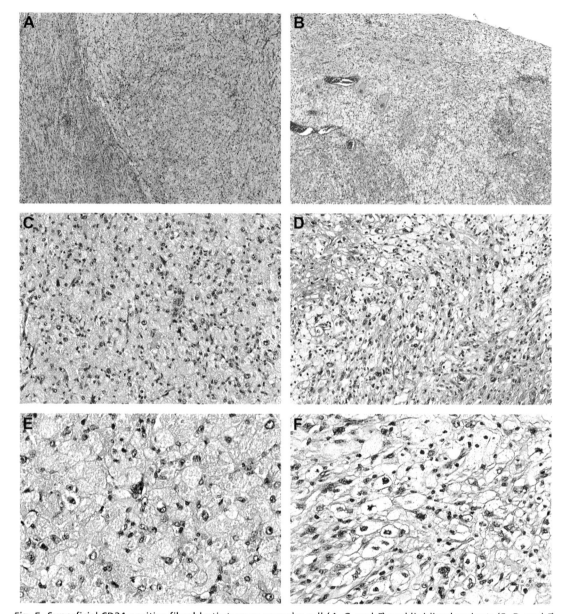

Fig. 5. Superficial CD34-positive fibroblastic tumor: granular cell (*A, C,* and *E*) and lipidized variants (*B, D,* and *F*).

Superficial CD34-positive fibroblastic tumor does not harbor significant unbalanced chromosomal aberrations or recurrent gene variants (see **Fig. 9**).[2,12] The former contrasts with pleomorphic sarcomas, which typically show complex karyotypes.

DIFFERENTIAL DIAGNOSIS

Due to its broad morphologic spectrum, the differential diagnosis of CD34FT is wide-ranging and includes benign, intermediate malignancy, and overtly malignant neoplasms (sarcomas). Hereafter, we will mention the main clinical,

morphologic, immunohistochemical, and molecular features which allow the distinction of entities that fall in the differential of CD34FT.

SARCOMAS

- Pleomorphic sarcomas (*myxofibrosarcoma, leiomyosarcoma, liposarcoma and undifferentiated pleomorphic sarcoma*): typically affect older adults (>60 year old) and generally show infiltrative borders. Furthermore, except for myxofibrosarcoma, most pleomorphic sarcomas originate in the deep soft tissues of the

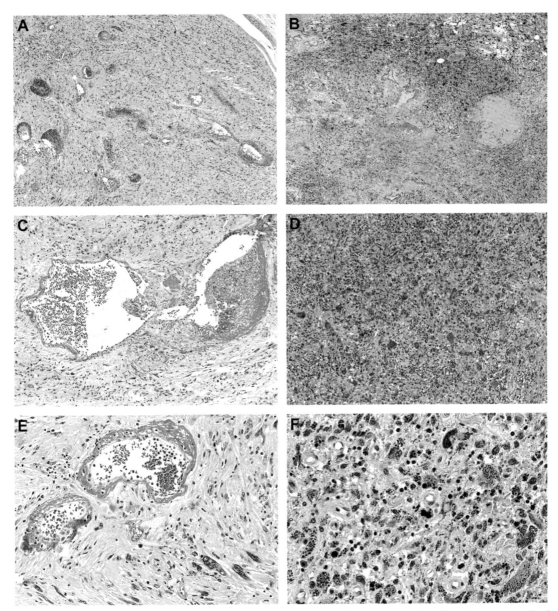

Fig. 6. Pleomorphic hyalinizing angiectatic tumor-like variant of superficial CD34-positive fibroblastic tumor (*A-F*).

extremities. On histology, they are generally densely cellular, show brisk mitotic activity and present areas of necrosis. On immunohistochemistry, CD34 is rarely expressed in undifferentiated pleomorphic sarcoma and leiomyosarcoma, but can be positive in liposarcoma and myxofibrosarcoma, albeit in a more focal and less intense manner than CD34FT.

- Epithelioid sarcoma: both proximal and distal variants generally present as poorly circumscribed masses composed of epithelioid to spindle cells which generally lack significant nuclear pleomorphism. Necrosis is common, but mitotic activity can be low. On immunohistochemistry, ~50% are focally to diffusely positive with CD34 and most express epithelial markers (pan-keratin and EMA), usually strongly and diffusely. Finally, the vast majority of epithelioid sarcomas (~95% of cases) show loss of SMARCB1 (INI-1) nuclear expression.

INTERMEDIATE MALIGNANCY TUMORS

- Pseudomyogenic hemangioendothelioma: in most cases (~60%) this tumor is multifocal and often involves multiple tissue planes. Most cases are composed of spindle to

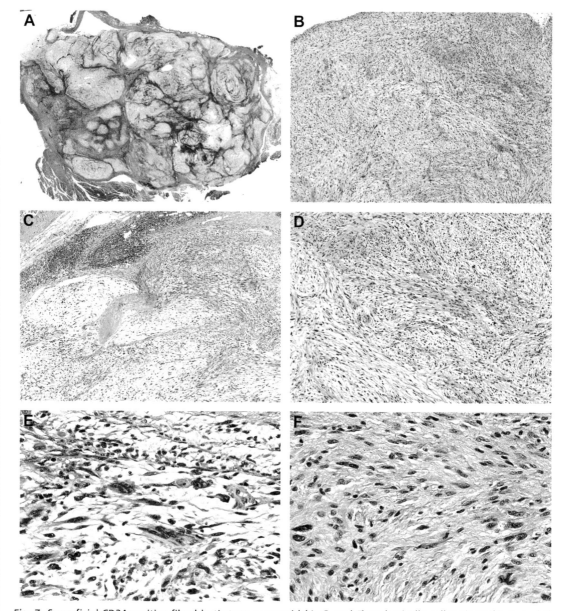

Fig. 7. Superficial CD34-positive fibroblastic tumor: myxoid (*A, C,* and *E*) and spindle cell variants (*B, D,* and *F*).

epithelioid cells, similar to the cells of CD34FT, but nuclear pleomorphism is a rare finding. On immunohistochemistry, they are positive for ERG, pan-keratin, and FOSB,[14] but generally do not express CD34. Finally, pseudomyogenic hemangioendothelioma shows recurrent *FOSB* rearrangements.[15]

- Pleomorphic hyalinizing angiectatic tumor (PHAT): it can be extremely challenging to distinguish PHAT from CD34FT to the point that in several studies, a subset of CD34FT was originally classified as PHAT (even by expert soft tissue pathologists).[1,2,4,8]

Compared to CD34FT, prototypical cases of PHAT are more infiltrative, show a prominent component of ectatic blood vessels with fibrinous walls, which are generally homogeneously distributed across the tumor surface, and neoplastic cells rarely have abundant and brightly eosinophilic cytoplasm. In addition, a component made of spindle cells lacking significant pleomorphism and with variable hemosiderin deposits is frequently encountered in the periphery of PHAT. On immunohistochemistry, CD34 is focal to diffusely positive in ~50% of cases

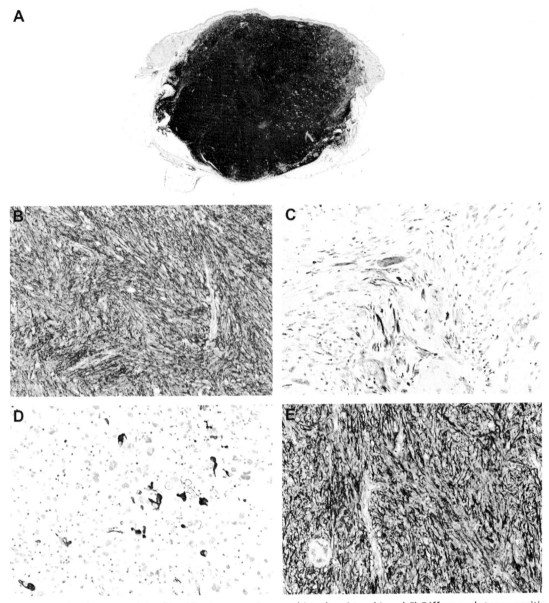

Fig. 8. Superficial CD34-positive fibroblastic tumor: immunohistochemistry. (*A* and *B*) Diffuse and strong positivity of CD34. (*C*) Focal patchy expression of pan-keratin (AE1-AE3). (*D*) Focal patchy expression of desmin. (*E*) Diffuse and strong expression of SynCAM3.

of PHAT, while pan-keratin is negative. Finally, PHAT shows recurrent *TGFBR3* and *OGA* gene rearrangements,[16] which have never been demonstrated in CD34FT.[1,9]

- Myxoinflammatory fibroblastic sarcoma: most cases occur in the distal extremities (hands, wrists, ankle, and foot), are vaguely multinodular and infiltrate the deep fascial planes. Myxoid stromal changes are more frequently present than in CD34FT and sometimes alternate with poorly cellular hyaline areas. On immunohistochemistry, CD34 is positive in ~50% of cases but rarely as

strongly and diffusely as in CD34FT. From a molecular standpoint, myxoinflammatory fibroblastic sarcoma has complex structural alterations (*VGLL3* amplification, *TGFBR3*/*OGA* rearrangements, *BRAF* fusion/amplification) and, in rare cases, *YAP1::MAML2* gene fusions.[17–19]

- Solitary fibrous tumor: composed predominantly of monomorphic spindle cells associated with a rich vasculature of ramified blood vessels that sometimes have thick hyalinized walls. In rare instances, nuclear pleomorphism can be present and may complicate the

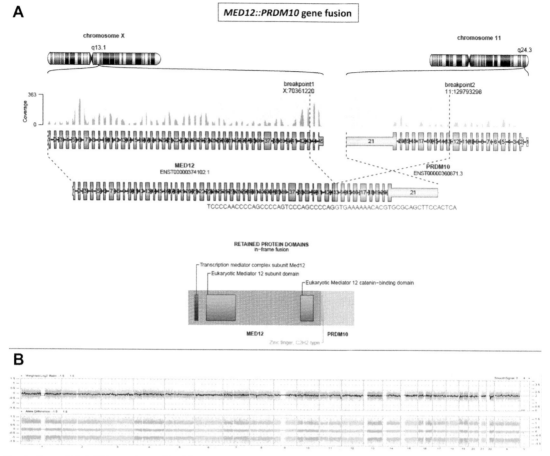

Fig. 9. Superficial CD34-Positive fibroblastic tumor: molecular and cytogenetic features. (*A*) Schematic representations of the loci of *MED12* (NM_005120.3) in Xq13.1 and *PRDM10* (NM_199437.2) in 11q24.3, a *MED12::PRDM10* gene fusion and its putative chimeric protein. (*B*) Array-comparative genomic hybridization (aCGH) profile showing a "silent profile" lacking significant copy number gains or losses. Chromosomes 1 to X/Y are plotted on the x-axis and copy number alterations on the y-axis. (Image Courtesy Figure (*A*) *Rihab Azmani PhD*.)

differential with CD34FT.[20] On immunohistochemistry, solitary fibrous tumor is diffusely and strongly positive with CD34 (>90% of cases) but does not express keratins. In challenging cases (ie, core needle biopsies), STAT6 can prove helpful as it is positive in virtually all cases of solitary fibrous tumors due to recurrent *NAB2::STAT6* gene fusions.[21]

- Dermatofibrosarcoma protuberans: in contrast to CD34FT, these tumors are composed of monomorphic spindle cells and have infiltrative borders. On immunohistochemistry, CD34 is diffusely and strongly expressed in most cases, but, in contrast to CD34FT, keratins are consistently negative.

BENIGN TUMORS

- Deep fibrous histiocytoma: composed predominantly of uniform spindle cells arranged in a storiform pattern. Around 40% of cases express CD34, while keratins are negative.
- Granular cell tumor and "non-neural granular cell tumor": these tumors have ill-defined borders and are typically entirely composed of epithelioid cells with abundant eosinophilic and granular cytoplasm. Classic granular cell tumor is diffusely and strongly positive with S100 and SOX10, while "non-neural granular cell tumor" is generally positive with ALK and negative for CD34 and keratins.[22,23]

PROGNOSIS AND MANAGEMENT

Superficial CD34-positive fibroblastic tumor is classified as an "intermediate malignancy tumor" per current World Health Organization criteria.[24] Based on the published series (see **Box 1**), the risk for local recurrence seems to be low (~9% of cases), and metastatic spread (to regional

Table 1
Frequency of expression of selected immunohistochemical markers in Superficial CD34-positive fibroblastic tumor

Marker	Frequency of Expression % (range)	Pattern of Expression	Number of Cases
CD34	100%	cytoplasmic, diffuse and strong intensity	132
Pan-keratin (AE1-AE3)	74% (40%–100%)	cytoplasmic, focal or multifocal	81
Smooth muscle actin	8% (0%–13%)	cytoplasmic, focal	82
Desmin	30% (0%–57%)	cytoplasmic, focal to multifocal	102
SynCAM3	95% (95%–100%)	cytoplasmic, diffuse, moderate to strong intensity	119
WT1	75%	nuclear, focal to diffuse	52
PRDM10	50% (40%–53%)	nuclear, focal to diffuse	18
Cyclin D1	100%	nuclear and cytoplasmic, diffuse	5
MDM2	83%	nuclear, focal to multifocal	12
S100	0%	-	34
ERG	0%	-	16
ALK	0%	-	18
H-Caldesmon	0%	-	7

References: Carter and colleagues[1]; Perret and colleagues[2]; Puls and colleagues[4,5]; Lao and colleagues[6]; Anderson and colleagues[8]; Zhao and colleagues[10]; Sugita and colleagues[13]

lymph nodes) has been only exceptionally reported (~2% of cases). Despite the rare cases showing metastatic spread to regional lymph nodes, no disease-associated deaths have been reported. It is, however, important to remark that only a small proportion of published cases (18/99, 18%) had long-term follow-up (>5 years). Concerning management, as with most intermediate malignancy tumors, the primary treatment of CD34FT is surgical excision with negative margins; there is no evidence of the utility of radiotherapy or chemotherapy.

Table 2
Gene fusions reported in Superficial CD34-positive fibroblastic tumor

5′ Gene (exon)	3′ Gene (exon)	N° of Cases
MED12 (42 or 43)	PRDM10 (13 or 14)	16
CITED2 (2)	PRDM10 (14)	5
PRDM10 (11)	RAB30 (3)	1
PRDM10 (13)	ARHGAP32 (5)	1

References: Perret and colleagues[2]; Puls and colleagues[4,5]; Zhao and colleagues[10]

CLINICS CARE POINTS

- Superficial CD34-positive fibroblastic tumor is a distinctive low grade neoplasm that shows a deceiving histomorphology, mimicking pleomorphic sarcomas.

- Ensuring the correct diagnosis of superficial CD34-positive fibroblastic tumor is vital in order to avoid unnecessary adjuvant treatment.

- The combination of meticulous assessment of clinical and histomorphological features and a limited panel of widely available immunohistochemical markers is enough to obtain an accurate diagnosis in most cases.

DISCLOSURE

The authors have nothing to disclose.

ACKNOWLEDGMENTS

The authors wish to thank the following colleagues for kindly providing detailed information about their studies on superficial CD34-positive fibroblastic tumor: Professor Christopher D.M. Fletcher (Boston, MA), Dr William J. Anderson (Boston, MA) and Dr Florian Puls (Gothenburg, Sweden). We also wish to thank Rihab Azmani PhD for providing **Fig. 9**A and all members of the French sarcoma network (RRePS).

REFERENCES

1. Carter JM, Weiss SW, Linos K, et al. Superficial CD34-positive fibroblastic tumor: Report of 18 cases of a distinctive low-grade mesenchymal neoplasm of intermediate (borderline) malignancy. Mod Pathol 2014;27(2):294–302.
2. Perret R, Michal M, Carr RA, et al. Superficial CD34-positive fibroblastic tumor and PRDM10-rearranged soft tissue tumor are overlapping entities: a comprehensive study of 20 cases. Histopathology 2021;79(5):810–25.
3. Batur S, Ozcan K, Ozcan G, et al. Superficial CD34 positive fibroblastic tumor: report of three cases and review of the literature. Int J Dermatol 2019;58(4):416–22.
4. Puls F, Pillay N, Fagman H, et al. PRDM10-rearranged Soft Tissue Tumor: A Clinicopathologic Study of 9 Cases. Am J Surg Pathol 2018;43(4):504–13.
5. Puls F, Carter JM, Pillay N, et al. Overlapping morphological, immunohistochemical and genetic features of superficial CD34-positive fibroblastic tumor and PRDM10-rearranged soft tissue tumor. Mod Pathol an Off J United States Can Acad Pathol Inc 2022;35(6):767–76.
6. Lao IW, Yu L, Wang J. Superficial CD34-positive fibroblastic tumour: a clinicopathological and immunohistochemical study of an additional series. Histopathology 2017;70(3):394–401.
7. Hendry SA, Wong DD, Papadimitriou J, et al. Superficial CD34-positive fibroblastic tumour: report of two new cases. Pathology 2015;47(5):479–82.
8. Anderson WJ, Mertens F, Mariño-Enríquez A, et al. Superficial CD34-Positive Fibroblastic Tumor: A Clinicopathologic, Immunohistochemical, and Molecular Study of 59 Cases. Am J Surg Pathol 2022;46(10):1329–39.
9. Ding L, Xu W-J, Tao X-Y, et al. Clinicopathological features of superficial CD34-positive fibroblastic tumor. World J Clin cases 2021;9(12):2739–50.
10. Zhao M, Yin X, He H, et al. Recurrent PRDM10 Fusions in Superficial CD34-Positive Fibroblastic Tumors : A Clinicopathologic and Molecular Study of 10 Additional Cases of an Emerging Novel Entity. Am J Clin Pathol 2023;159(4):367–78.
11. Mao X, Sun Y, Deng M, et al. Superficial CD34-positive fibroblastic tumor : report of two cases and review of literature. Int J Clin Exp 2020;13(1):38–43.
12. Hofvander J, Puls F, Pillay N, et al. Undifferentiated pleomorphic sarcomas with PRDM10 fusions have a distinct gene expression profile. J Pathol 2019;249(4):425–34.
13. Sugita S, Takenami T, Kido T, et al. Usefulness of SynCAM3 and cyclin D1 immunohistochemistry in distinguishing superficial CD34-positive fibroblastic tumor from its histological mimics. Med Mol Morphol 2023;56(1):69–77.
14. Hung YP, Fletcher CDM, Hornick JL. FOSB is a Useful Diagnostic Marker for Pseudomyogenic Hemangioendothelioma. Am J Surg Pathol 2017;41(5):596–606.
15. Walther C, Tayebwa J, Lilljebjörn H, et al. A novel SERPINE1-FOSB fusion gene results in transcriptional up-regulation of FOSB in pseudomyogenic haemangioendothelioma. J Pathol 2014;232(5):534–40.
16. Carter JM, Sukov WR, Montgomery E, et al. TGFBR3 and MGEA5 rearrangements in pleomorphic hyalinizing angiectatic tumors and the spectrum of related neoplasms. Am J Surg Pathol 2014;38(9):1182–92.
17. Kao YC, Ranucci V, Zhang L, et al. Recurrent BRAF Gene Rearrangements in Myxoinflammatory Fibroblastic Sarcomas, but Not Hemosiderotic Fibrolipomatous Tumors. Am J Surg Pathol 2017;41(11):1456–65.
18. Perret R, Tallegas M, Velasco V, et al. Recurrent YAP1::MAML2 fusions in "nodular necrotizing" variants of myxoinflammatory fibroblastic sarcoma: a comprehensive study of 7 cases. Mod Pathol an Off J United States Can Acad Pathol Inc 2022;35(10):1398–404.
19. Antonescu CR, Zhang L, Nielsen GP, et al. Consistent t(1;10) with rearrangements of TGFBR3 and MGEA5 in both myxoinflammatory fibroblastic sarcoma and hemosiderotic fibrolipomatous tumor. Genes Chromosomes Cancer 2011;50(10):757–64.
20. Demicco EG, Park MS, Araujo DM, et al. Solitary fibrous tumor: a clinicopathological study of 110 cases and proposed risk assessment model. Mod Pathol an Off J United States Can Acad Pathol Inc 2012;25(9):1298–306.
21. Doyle LA, Vivero M, Fletcher CD, et al. Nuclear expression of STAT6 distinguishes solitary fibrous tumor from histologic mimics. Mod Pathol an Off J United States Can Acad Pathol Inc 2014;27(3):390–5.
22. Cohen JN, Yeh I, Jordan RC, et al. Cutaneous Non-Neural Granular Cell Tumors Harbor Recurrent ALK Gene Fusions. Am J Surg Pathol 2018;42(9):1133–42.
23. Perret RE, Jullie M-L, Vergier B, et al. A subset of so-called dermal non-neural granular cell tumours are underlined by ALK fusions, further supporting the idea that they represent a variant of epithelioid fibrous histiocytoma. Histopathology 2018;73(3):532–4.
24. WHO Classification of Tumours Editorial Board. WHO classification of tumours of soft tissue and bone. 5th edition. Lyon, France: IARC Press; 2020.

GLI1-Altered Mesenchymal Tumors

Jeffrey M. Cloutier, MD, PhD[a,b], Darcy A. Kerr, MD[a,b],*

KEYWORDS

• *GLI1* • Fusion • Amplified • Mesenchymal tumor • Glomoid neoplasm • Pericytoma

---

Key points

- *GLI1*-altered mesenchymal tumors are an emerging category of neoplasms with fusions or amplifications of *GLI1*.
- They occur across a broad age range and diverse anatomic sites, often involving the head and neck.
- They are typically multinodular tumors composed of nests of uniform round-to-ovoid cells with a rich vascular network and an inconsistent immunophenotype.
- Recent evidence indicates that they have the potential to metastasize.

ABSTRACT

GLI1-altered mesenchymal tumors comprise an emerging group of neoplasms characterized by fusions or amplifications involving *GLI1*, a gene that encodes a key regulator of the Hedgehog signaling pathway. In recent years, tumors with GLI1 alterations have been reported across a variety of anatomic sites and a broad age range. Although these tumors can exhibit a wide morphologic spectrum and a variable immunophenotype, they frequently present with monomorphic ovoid cells arranged in distinctive nests with a rich, arborizing vascular network. Recent evidence indicates that they have the potential to metastasize, which suggests that they may be best considered a sarcoma.

OVERVIEW

Fusions or amplifications involving the *GLI1* gene have been identified in mesenchymal tumors exhibiting diverse morphology, immunophenotypes, and clinical characteristics. In 2004, Dahlén and colleagues first described a distinctive group of soft tissue tumors harboring *ACTB::GLI1* fusions mediated by a t(7;12) translocation.[1] These tumors, which arose in the tongue, stomach, and calf, were characterized by a lobulated proliferation of uniform ovoid cells, a prominent thin-walled vascular network, and co-expression of smooth muscle actin and laminin. Based on these features and ultrastructural characteristics, they were thought to fall on the spectrum of myopericytic/pericytic neoplasms, and the name "pericytoma with t(7;12)" was proposed.

Since then, numerous other *GLI1*-rearranged tumors have been reported at various anatomic sites, including the head and neck with a predilection for the tongue,[2–5] various soft tissue sites,[2,6–8] bone,[2,9,10] gastrointestinal tract,[11,12] genitourinary tract (kidney),[13,14] gynecologic tract (ovary and uterus),[9,14–17] intrathoracic sites,[18] and retroperitoneum.[2] *GLI1* rearrangements are also found in two histologically distinctive and well-characterized gastric neoplasms that typically occur in young patients, plexiform fibromyxoma and gastroblastoma, both of which harbor *MALAT1::GLI1* fusions.[19,20]

---

[a] Department of Pathology and Laboratory Medicine, Dartmouth-Hitchcock Medical Center, 1 Medical Center Drive, Lebanon, NH 03756, USA; [b] Dartmouth Geisel School of Medicine, 1 Rope Ferry Road, Hanover, NH 03755, USA
* Corresponding author.
E-mail address: Darcy.A.Kerr@hitchcock.org
Twitter: @JCloutierMD (J.M.C.); @darcykerrMD (D.A.K.)

Surgical Pathology 17 (2024) 13–24
https://doi.org/10.1016/j.path.2023.06.004
1875-9181/24/© 2023 Elsevier Inc. All rights reserved.

surgpath.theclinics.com

The remaining *GLI1*-rearranged tumors exhibit notable morphologic similarities. While these lesions share some histologic features with pericytoma, including uniform round-to-ovoid cell morphology, nested architecture, and a rich vascular network, they exhibit more morphologic variability and overall have shown inconsistent immunoreactivity for actin, raising questions about their true line of differentiation.

In addition to *GLI1* fusions, recent studies have identified high-level gene amplifications involving *GLI1* in tumors with significant morphologic overlap with *GLI1*-fusion-positive tumors.[14,21,22] These tumors typically also show co-amplification of several neighboring genes located in the 12q13-q15 region.[21] These neoplasms have exhibited a spectrum of histologic features and an inconsistent immunohistochemical profile, yet they show sufficient overlap with *GLI1*-rearranged mesenchymal tumors to suggest that they are likely pathogenetically related.

The term "*GLI1*-altered mesenchymal tumor" has been recently proposed for this collective group of neoplasms with similar morphologic features and fusions or amplifications of *GLI1*.[23] Similarly, the term "*GLI1*-altered soft tissue tumor" is used in the current (5th edition) WHO classification of head and neck tumors.[24] Although the initial cases of "pericytoma with t(7;12)" showed indolent clinical behavior, there have since been several reports of *GLI1*-rearranged and amplified tumors giving rise to locoregional and distant metastases.[2,6,9,14,21,25] Despite ongoing research, it remains unclear whether this category represents a singular clinicopathologic entity or a heterogeneous group of soft tissue neoplasms with frequent *GLI1* alterations. While the precise classification and etiologic nature of these tumors is an evolving topic, their potential to metastasize indicates that classifying them as sarcomas might be appropriate. This review aims to highlight the current clinicopathologic and molecular understanding of *GLI1*-altered mesenchymal tumors.

CLINICAL PRESENTATION

GLI1-altered mesenchymal tumors tend to present in younger to middle-aged adults, with a median age of approximately 38 years. However, the reported age range is broad (1–88 years). In several cases, tumors have developed in infants and children, including one that presented congenitally in the tongue.[11,15,21–23,26,27] While one study found that *GLI1*-amplified tumors may occur in slightly older patients,[3] analysis of all reported cases to date reveals that both *GLI1*-amplified and *GLI1*-fusion-positive cases exhibit a comparable median age (35 vs 38 years). There does not appear to be a significant sex predilection, with males and females affected roughly equally.

Tumors may arise at diverse anatomic sites. Most reported cases have involved soft tissue, while primary bone tumors are rare. About one-third of all reported cases have occurred in the head and neck region, with the tongue being particularly susceptible, accounting for approximately 70% of these cases.[1,2,4,5,21–23,27–29] Tumors also frequently present in deep soft tissue of the extremities and trunk.[1,2,7,8,21,23,26,27] Tumors less commonly occur in visceral organs, including the tubular gastrointestinal tract (stomach, jejunum, duodenum),[1,11,12,23,30,31] kidney,[13,14] and gynecologic tract (ovary, uterus, and uterine cervix),[9,14–17,23,32] as well as the intrathoracic and retroperitoneal spaces.[2,18] Primary osseous tumors have involved the talus, cervical spine, tibia, and scapula.[2,9,10] Rare cutaneous and subcutaneous cases have also been reported.[27,33,34]

The clinical presentation is variable depending upon the specific site of involvement. In general, the majority of cases appear to show slow painless growth, and tumors may be present for several years to a decade prior to diagnosis.[23,26,33] Osseous tumors may erode through the cortex and extend into soft tissue.[9] Ovarian or uterine involvement may be associated with symptoms of abdominal pain, bloating, and/or a palpable abdominal mass.[15,16]

GROSS FEATURES

Macroscopically, tumors are circumscribed, unencapsulated masses with a nodular or multinodular appearance (**Fig. 1**). The cut surface has been described as grey-white to yellow-brown, solid, partially solid and cystic, fleshy, and gelatinous. Areas of hemorrhage and rarely necrosis may be present. The median tumor size is 4 cm, with a range of 0.8 cm to 21 cm.

MICROSCOPIC FEATURES

GLI1-altered mesenchymal tumors usually exhibit a multinodular, lobulated, or plexiform architecture (**Fig. 2**). Lobules of tumor are frequently separated by thick fibrous bands. While the neoplasms are generally relatively well-circumscribed, they often demonstrate infiltration into adjacent tissues. Tumors are typically composed of monomorphic ovoid-to-round or vaguely epithelioid cells arranged in compact or ill-defined nests that are separated by a well-developed arborizing capillary network. Frequently, perivascular aggregates of tumor cells protrude into dilated vascular spaces,

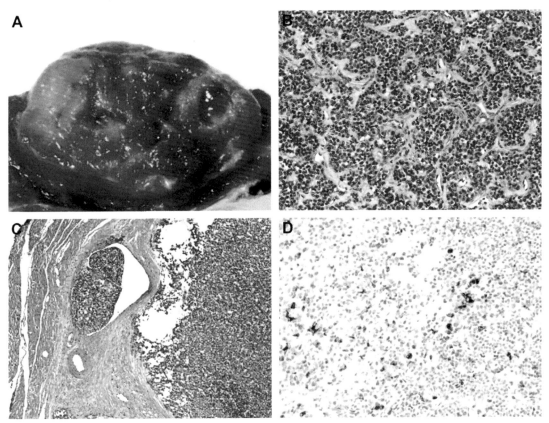

Fig. 1. Representative gross and microscopic images of a GLI1-fusion-positive mesechymal tumor occurring in the tibia. (A) Grossly, the tumors typically appear as well-circumscribed, nodular masses with a fleshy tan cut surface and foci of hemorrhage. (B) Microscopically, the tumor cells display a vaguely nested arrangement, composed of a monomophoic population of round-to-ovoid cells with a conspicuous vascular network. (C) Lymphovascular invasion is observed in some cases. (D) Tumors often have a non-specific immunophenotype. In this case, focal expression of synaptophysin was observed (an uncommon feature).

mimicking lymphovascular invasion. True vascular invasion has been identified in a subset of cases. Tumors typically have a dense fibrous stroma often with myxoid areas.

Cytologically, the tumor cells have uniform round-to-oval nuclei with fine to vesicular chromatin and small centrally located or inconspicuous nucleoli (**Figs. 3** and **4**). The cells exhibit limited to moderate amounts of cytoplasm, which is clear or pale-eosinophilic. Cytoplasmic vacuolization, resembling that seen in lipoblasts, is occasionally observed. Nuclear atypia or pleomorphism is generally absent, although rare cases with increased pleomorphism and atypia have been described.[12,16,21,33] Tumors exhibit variable mitotic rates, most commonly 1 to 2 mitotic figures per 10 high-power fields (HPF), but ranging from rare to greater than 30 mitotic figures per 10 HPF.[12,32] Tumor necrosis is not common, but has been observed in a subset of cases.

Perhaps the most common overall morphologic pattern in GLI1-altered mesenchymal tumors presents monomorphic round-to-ovoid cells with nested growth and perivascular proliferation. In one recent series, tumors with these morphologic features were designated as "distinctive nested glomoid neoplasms," distinguishing them as a distinct subset of GLI1-altered tumors.[27] Various less common architectural patterns have been described, such as solid, corded, reticular, trabecular, pseudoglandular, pseudopapillary, microcystic, and sieve-like patterns. Rarely, tumors may present with cellular fascicles of spindle cells or biphasic (round-to-ovoid and spindled) morphology.[1,4,5,12,16,21,23] Additionally, tumors may show prominent cystic change.

IMMUNOHISTOCHEMICAL FEATURES

The immunohistochemical profile of GLI1-altered mesenchymal tumors is variable and relatively non-specific (**Fig. 5**). While the original series of tumors described as "pericytoma with t(7;22)" were

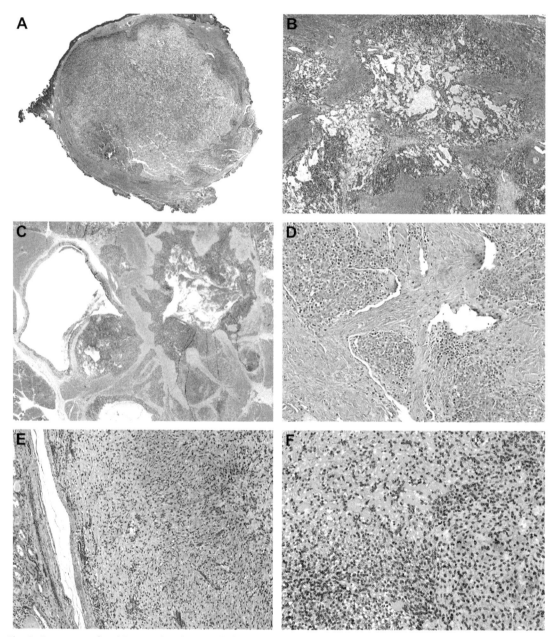

Fig. 2. Spectrum of architectural and stromal changes in *GLI1*-altered mesenchymal tumors. (*A*) Tumors are typically nodular or multinodular. (*B*) They often exhibit thick fibrous bands, myxoid change, and peripheral infiltration into adjacent tissues. (*C*) Occasionally, tumors may show prominent cystic change. (*D*) Subendothelial protrusions of tumor into vascular spaces is not infrequent and can mimic lymphovascular invasion in some cases. (*E*) *GLI1*-rearranged mesenchymal tumors can occur in various anatomic locations, as shown in this example of a kidney tumor with nodular growth and myxoid stromal change. (*F*) This tumor exhibited areas of dense stromal hyalinization between cords of tumor cells. All cases were positive for a *GLI1* fusion.

positive for smooth muscle actin (SMA),[1] subsequent studies have not found SMA to be consistently expressed in *GLI1*-altered tumors. CD56 is the most consistently expressed marker. The immunohistochemical expression of S100 protein has been observed in approximately half of cases to varying degrees, ranging from focal to diffuse.[2,22,23] By contrast, SOX10 is consistently negative.

In addition to CD56 reactivity, many cases have shown expression of another relatively nonspecific marker of neuroendocrine differentiation, NSE, while synaptophysin and chromogranin are

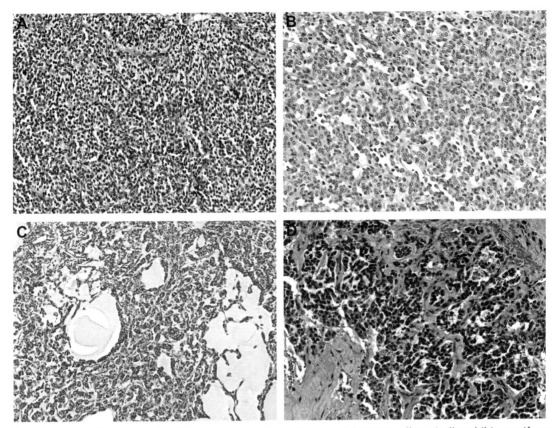

Fig. 3. Morphologic features of *GLI1*-altered mesenchymal tumors. (*A*) Tumor cells typically exhibit a uniform, round-to-ovoid- -morphology and are often arranged in distinct nests that are separated by a dense capillary network. (*B*) In some instances, tumors may display a solid growth pattern, lacking well-defined nests. (*C*) Tumors may exhibit a variety of patterns, including corded to reticular and cystic or sieve-like patterns, frequently in association with myxoid stroma. (*D*) Tumor cells typically display monomorphic nuclei with limited pleomorphism. All cases were positive for a *GLI1* fusion.

typically negative or only focal (see **Fig.** 1D).[4,7,10,11,17,18,21–23,26,29–31,33,34] Studies and case reports have demonstrated variable expression of a variety of other markers, including EMA, cyclin D1, CD10, BCL-2, BCOR, and D2-40.[4,12,14,16,17,23,26,27,29,31,33] Recently, strong and near diffuse p16 expression was documented in a subset of cases.[5,33] *GLI1*-altered mesenchymal tumors do not consistently express markers of myoepithelial (GFAP and calponin), vascular (ERG and CD31), or myogenic (desmin, myogenin, and MyoD1) differentiation. Keratins are also typically negative, with only a small subset of cases exhibiting focal keratin immunoreactivity.

Overexpression of adjacent co-amplified gene products, such as MDM2, STAT6, and CDK4, is commonly observed in cases with *GLI1* amplification.[5,14,21–23,33] Immunohistochemical expression of these markers may be a helpful clue toward the diagnosis of a *GLI1*-amplified tumor.

Recent work suggests that immunohistochemistry for GLI1 may serve as a useful ancillary tool for the diagnosis of *GLI1*-altered tumors.[12,33,35] In one recent study, Parrak and colleagues found that GLI1 immunohistochemical expression had a 91% sensitivity and 98% specificity for a diagnosis of *GLI1*-altered mesenchymal tumors, including both fusion and amplification-driven tumors.[35] GLI1 typically localizes to both the nucleus and cytoplasm (**Fig. 6**), but it may also be exclusively nuclear.[35]

MOLECULAR PATHOLOGY FEATURES

GLI1 (GLI family zinc finger 1 or glioma-associated oncogene homologue 1), located on chromosome 12q13.3, encodes a transcription factor of the Kruppel family of zinc finger proteins, which plays a critical role in the Hedgehog signaling pathway. *GLI1* gene fusions and amplifications lead to an increase in the expression of both *GLI1* mRNA

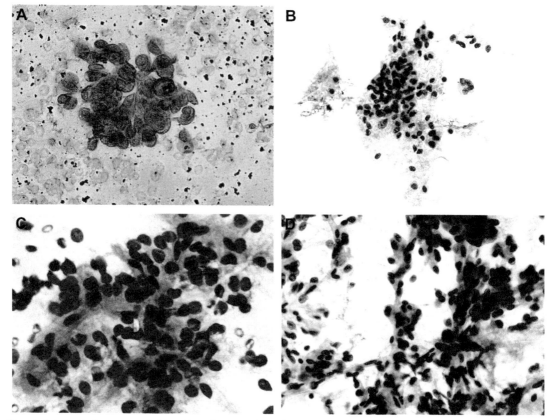

Fig. 4. Cytologic features of *GLI1*-altered mesenchymal tumors recapitulate the histologic features. (*A, B*) Example of a *GLI1*-amplified mesenchymal tumor showing (*A*) small round cells with scant cytoplasm and subtle nuclear molding on Giemsa stain and (*B*) a sheet-like configuration of cohesive round-to-ovoid cells on ThinPrep stain. (*C, D*) Example of a *GLI1*-fusion-positive mesenchymal tumor exhibiting (*C*) round-to-ovoid cells with a slightly fibrillary stroma on Giemsa stain and (*D*) a prominent background capillary vasculature on Pap stain. (Photo credits: Anthony W. Chi, MD, PhD (*A* and *B*), Wei-Lien Wang, MD (*C* and *D*).)

transcripts and protein, and subsequent activation of downstream targets with key roles in tumorigenesis.[2,19–21]

A significant number of *GLI1*-fusion-positive tumors are the result of fusions between the 5′ segment of *ACTB* and the 3′ segment of *GLI1*, leading to the formation of an *ACTB::GLI1* transcript.[1] However, the spectrum of *GLI1* fusions is broad and includes a growing list of 5′ partner genes, such as *MALAT1, PTCH1, APOD, DERA, SYT, NCOR2, HNRNPA1, TXNIP, NEAT*, and *PAMR1*.[2,7,8,16,22,23,27]

GLI1 fusions operate through a mechanism known as promoter swapping, in which the promoter region of *GLI1* is substituted with the highly active promoter region of the 5′ fusion partner. As a result, the expression of *GLI1* becomes deregulated, leading to abnormal mRNA and protein production. *GLI1* fusions typically occur within exons 4, 5, 6, or 7. These breakpoints lead to the retention of the functional FOXP coiled-coil and DNA-

binding zinc finger domains encoded by the 3′ portion of *GLI1*. Despite being truncated, the resulting protein retains its ability to activate downstream targets.[18,19] Meanwhile, the 5′ gene partner can have variable breakpoints that involve either exonic or intronic sequences. Although *GLI1* is the 3′ partner in most cases, there have been 2 documented cases in which *GLI1* acts as the 5′ fusion partner.[13,14] Interestingly, both tumors occurred in the kidney and were associated with a *GLI1::FOXO4* fusion. These tumors displayed slightly different morphologic features, including a non-nested growth pattern with a dense, hyalinized stroma separating tumor cells (see **Figs. 2**E-F). Currently, it is not clear whether these morphologic differences can be attributed to the variant fusions observed in these tumors.

GLI1-amplified tumors represent a molecularly distinct subset of *GLI1*-altered mesenchymal tumors (approximately one-third of reported cases), characterized by high-level amplification of

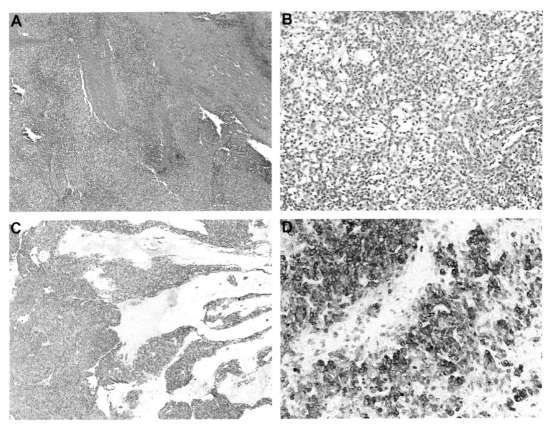

Fig. 5. Morphologic and immunohistochemical features of a *GLI1*-amplified mesenchymal tumor occurring in the tongue. (*A*) The tumor exhibits a solid growth pattern, with thick fibrous bands coursing through it. (*B*) In areas, the tumor cells show a slight reticular pattern with edematous stroma. The tumor cells are monomorphic and ovoid with even chromatin and minimal cytoplasm. (*C*) Many tumors are immunoreactive for CD56. (*D*) In addition, a subset of tumors shows immunoreactivity for S100 protein, which may be focal or diffuse. (Photo credits: Anthony W. Chi, MD, PhD.)

GLI1.[14,21–23,26,33] This *GLI1* amplification is frequently associated with co-amplification of nearby genes on 12q13-q15, such as *DDIT3*, *CDK4*, *MDM2*, *STAT6*, *HMGA2*, *LRP1*, *FRS2*, *ARHGEF25*, and/or *TSPAN31*.[21,23,26] Studies have demonstrated that this amplification can cause overexpression of the proteins produced by the amplified genes, which can be detected using immunohistochemistry. Given their close genomic proximity, FISH employing probes for *DDIT3*, *MDM2*, and *CDK4* may be particularly useful for the detection of *GLI1*-amplified tumors.[5,21,23,26,33] There have also been reports of rare cases that exhibit both copy number gain and evidence of a *GLI1* fusion.[21,23,27]

DIFFERENTIAL DIAGNOSIS

Diagnosing *GLI1*-altered mesenchymal neoplasms can be challenging due to their varied clinical, morphologic, and immunohistochemical characteristics, which can make the differential

diagnosis quite broad. In particular, myoepithelial neoplasms can exhibit strikingly similar features, including a predilection for the head and neck. They also share lobulated architecture, nested growth pattern, round-to-epithelioid morphology, clear cytoplasm, foci of myxoid stroma, and expression of S100 and/or SMA. The presence of a well-developed vascular network, subendothelial tumor proliferations, and lack of expression of other myoepithelial markers, such as keratins, SOX10, GFAP, and calponin, would favor *GLI1*-altered mesenchymal tumor. Difficult cases may be resolved with molecular testing. Of note, there has been a single case report of a tumor harboring a *TUBA1A::GLI1* fusion, which exhibited co-expression of keratin, S100, SOX10, and GFAP, and was therefore interpreted as more likely to represent a true myoepithelial neoplasm.[6]

Differentiating a *GLI1*-altered mesenchymal tumor from cellular glomus tumor or myopericytoma may be especially challenging to at times impossible, particularly when SMA positivity is present.

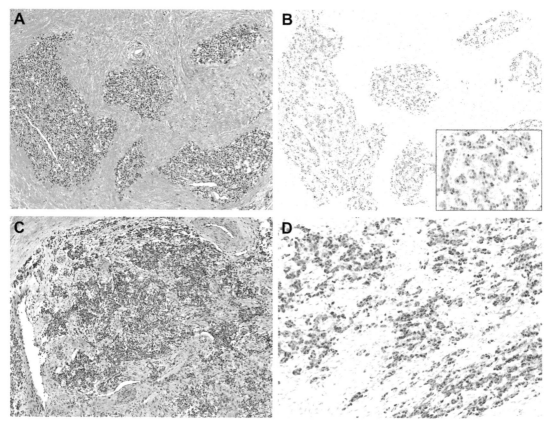

Fig. 6. Immunohistochemistry for GLI1 is a helpful diagnostic tool for identifying *GLI1*-altered mesenchymal tumors. (*A*) Representative histopathologic image of a tumor classified as "distinctive nested glomoid neoplasm," showing islands of nested monomorphic tumor cells separated by fibrous bands. (*B*) Corresponding immunohistochemical staining of the tumor with diffuse positivity for GLI1, showing nuclear and cytoplasmic localization (inset). (*C*) Representative histopathological image of a tumor classified as "pericytoma with t(7;12)," exhibiting irregular nests and islands of tumor cells in a fibrotic stroma. (*D*) Corresponding GLI1 immunohistochemical stain showing diffuse positivity in the tumor cells. (Photo credits: David J. Papke Jr., MD, PhD.)

In such cases, molecular testing may be necessary to make a distinction. Myopericytomas, glomus tumors, and angioleiomyomas are characterized by recurrent *PDGFB* and *NOTCH3* mutations, allowing for their genetic distinction from *GLI1*-altered mesenchymal tumors.[36,37]

It is worth noting that the nomenclature used to describe *GLI1*-altered mesenchymal tumors and their relationship to myopericytic/pericytic tumors is not without controversy. Some authors still classify tumors as t(7;12) pericytomas,[35] while others believe that most of these tumors are not truly pericytic in nature.[2] In fact, the current (5th edition) WHO classification of head and neck tumors does not recommend the use of the term "pericytoma" due to the lack of consistent criteria for these tumors.[24] This highlights the evolving nature of this area and the need for continued research to better understand the pathogenesis and classification of these tumors.

The nested growth pattern and frequent expression of CD56 and NSE may lead to a diagnostic consideration of paraganglioma or neuroendocrine tumor. Immunohistochemistry for synaptophysin and chromogranin can help to differentiate these neoplasms, as *GLI1*-altered tumors typically do not express these markers.

GLI1-altered mesenchymal tumors may also exhibit similarities with the recently described "pseudoendocrine sarcoma," including a lobulated architecture with fibrous septa, nested growth pattern of monomorphic ovoid cells, and occasional expression of S100. In general, these tumors may be distinguished on the basis of nuclear expression of beta-catenin, which is observed in the majority of cases of pseudoendocrine sarcoma.[38]

For cases presenting with a vaguely round cell morphology, the differential diagnosis could include Ewing sarcoma, other round cell sarcomas, and rhabdomyosarcoma. These tumors can generally be distinguished on the basis of immunohistochemistry or molecular testing. Strong and diffuse expression of membranous CD99 should distinguish most cases of Ewing sarcoma. Ewing sarcoma will typically also stain positively for NKX2.2 (negative in the few *GLI1*-altered mesenchymal tumors tested thus far[33]) and PAX7. Confirmatory molecular testing for an *EWSR1* or *FUS* rearrangement could be performed on cases that remain ambiguous after immunohistochemistry. Immunohistochemistry for desmin, MyoD1, and myogenin can be performed to exclude rhabdomyosarcoma.

Tumors manifesting S100 immunoreactivity may invoke a differential diagnosis that includes melanoma, clear cell sarcoma, and epithelioid schwannoma. SOX10, HMB-45, and Melan A can be performed to exclude these entities, as they are typically negative in *GLI1*-altered tumors. Of note, very rare cases with focal Melan A immunoreactivity have been documented.[13,32] While extraskeletal myxoid chondrosarcoma may show significant morphologic overlap with *GLI1*-rearranged tumors, these tumors harbor a characteristic *NR4A3* gene fusion. Alveolar soft part sarcoma could potentially resemble *GLI1*-rearranged tumors, with both showing a nested growth pattern and a thin-walled vascular network; however, they are distinguishable by their larger, more polygonal cells with dense eosinophilic cytoplasm and often prominent nucleoli, and their frequent positivity for PAS and TFE3. Of note, while the term "epithelioid" is not infrequently applied in the morphologic descriptions of *GLI1*-altered mesenchymal tumors, reported *GLI1*-altered tumors have lacked well-developed epithelioid morphology (ie, intermediate-to-large polyhedral cells with moderate-to-abundant cytoplasm).

GLI1-altered tumors that develop in the uterus may be mistaken for low-grade endometrial stroma sarcoma, whereas those arising in the ovary may be misinterpreted as primary ovarian tumors, such as sex cord stromal tumors. A panel of immunohistochemical markers, such as WT1, ER, PR, inhibin, SF1, and calretinin, can help to rule out these tumors. Notably, CD10 and cyclin D1 immunoreactivity has been reported in a subset of *GLI1*-altered cases, making these markers less useful for distinguishing *GLI1*-altered tumors in this differential diagnosis.[1,9,12,14,15,23]

Immunoreactivity for MDM2 and STAT6 in *GLI1*-amplified tumors can create potential pitfalls, leading to possible consideration of dedifferentiated liposarcoma and solitary fibrous tumor, respectively. Most cases of dedifferentiated liposarcoma occur in the retroperitoneum, which is a relatively uncommon site for *GLI1*-amplified tumors, and they often present with a well-differentiated component radiographically and histologically that allows for their distinction. Solitary fibrous tumors may be distinguished on the basis of strong and diffuse CD34 immunoreactivity, which is consistently negative in *GLI1*-altered mesenchymal tumors.

An increasing number of entities are defined by and named for their underlying molecular alterations. However, when interpreting molecular results, it is essential to keep in mind that certain alterations may not be specific to a particular disease. For instance, *GLI1* alterations are not disease-defining and can be observed in tumors of different lineages, including a subset of gliomas, alveolar rhabdomyosarcomas, osteosarcomas, and some carcinomas.[39–43] It is important to consider the clinical, morphologic, and immunohistochemical findings in conjunction with molecular results to make an accurate diagnosis of *GLI1*-altered mesenchymal tumor.

Recurrent *GLI1* fusions have been identified in two distinct types of gastric tumors, plexiform fibromyxoma, and gastroblastoma.[19,20,30] Plexiform fibromyxoma is a benign neoplasm that typically arises in the antrum or pyloric region, exhibiting a multinodular and plexiform architecture with uniform spindle cell morphology and SMA positivity. These tumors typically harbor *MALAT1::GLI1* fusions or *GLI1* polysomy, and despite exhibiting morphologic and immunohistochemical overlap with other *GLI1*-altered mesenchymal tumors, they are currently considered a distinct clinicopathologic entity.

Gastroblastoma, on the other hand, is a biphasic tumor with metastatic potential that typically presents in the gastric antrum with a male predilection and recurrent *MALAT1::GLI1* fusions.[20] These tumors are characterized by a biphasic proliferation of uniform spindle cells and nested epithelial cells. In contrast to other *GLI1*-altered mesenchymal tumors, gastroblastomas characteristically label for keratins, highlighting the epithelial component. Due to their distinctive clinicopathologic features, gastroblastomas are considered a separate entity from other *GLI1*-altered mesenchymal tumors.

PROGNOSIS

GLI1-altered mesenchymal tumors appear to behave similarly to low-grade to intermediate-grade sarcomas. Based on the currently reported cases with available clinical follow-up data, approximately 38% of patients developed a locoregional recurrence or distant metastasis.[2,9,12,14,16,21,23,27,29,32,33] Tumor recurrences may occur after incomplete excision of the primary tumor or there may be a period of many years between excision of the primary tumor and recurrence.[9,12,27] Metastases have been reported to involve lymph nodes, lungs, distant soft tissue sites, bone, liver, and brain.[2,9,12,14,16,21,29] At least two tumor-related deaths have been reported, both in patients with primary uterine tumors. Both tumors showed a spindle cell component, and one was a frankly morphologically malignant tumor (considered a uterine sarcoma).[14,16] High mitotic index, tumor necrosis, and high-grade morphology may correlate with poor outcomes.[2,14,16,21–23] However, metastases have also been documented in tumors with low mitotic rates and no necrosis, including those with typical nested architecture and bland cytomorphology,[9,25,29,30] despite a recent report suggesting that the nested pattern may be associated with indolent behavior.[38] The specific underlying molecular alteration (particular *GLI1* fusion partner or presence of *GLI1*-fusion vs *GLI1*-amplification) does not appear to correlate with prognosis. Ultimately, additional data is needed to inform appropriate risk stratification for patients with *GLI1*-altered mesenchymal tumors.

SUMMARY

GLI1-altered mesenchymal tumors are a group of neoplasms with malignant potential that share a common molecular signature characterized by gene fusions or amplifications involving *GLI1*. These tumors can show diverse clinical presentations and a broad spectrum of morphologic and immunohistochemical findings. Accurate diagnosis requires recognition of their distinctive histologic features, including frequent nested growth pattern, uniform round-to-ovoid cells, and rich capillary network, in combination with a thorough panel of immunohistochemical markers to exclude potential mimickers. These tumors frequently display a relatively monotonous cytomorphologic appearance typical of fusion-driven mesenchymal tumors. Molecular tools are useful to confirm the diagnosis.

CLINICS CARE POINTS

- *GLI1*-altered mesenchymal tumors represent a group of pathogenetically related neoplasms with fusions or amplifications of *GLI1*.
- Tumors may present across a broad age range, including infants and children, and occur at diverse anatomic sites, with frequent involvement of soft tissues and the head and neck.
- Tumors are typically multinodular, composed of nests of uniform round-to-ovoid cells separated by a rich thin-walled vascular network and fibrous bands.
- Immunophenotype is inconsistent, including frequent CD56 positivity and variable expression of SMA and S100 in a subset.
- Recent evidence has shown that *GLI1*-altered mesenchymal tumors are capable of metastasizing and thus may be best classified as a sarcoma.

DISCLOSURE

The authors have no conflicts of interest to declare.

REFERENCES

1. Dahlén A, Fletcher CDM, Mertens F, et al. Activation of the GLI oncogene through fusion with the beta-actin gene (ACTB) in a group of distinctive pericytic neoplasms: pericytoma with t(7;12). Am J Pathol 2004;164(5):1645–53.
2. Antonescu CR, Agaram NP, Sung YS, et al. A Distinct Malignant Epithelioid Neoplasm With GLI1 Gene Rearrangements, Frequent S100 Protein Expression, and Metastatic Potential: Expanding the Spectrum of Pathologic Entities With ACTB/MALAT1/PTCH1-GLI1 Fusions. Am J Surg Pathol 2018;42(4):553–60.
3. Xu B, Rasheed MRHA, Antonescu CR, et al. Pan-Trk immunohistochemistry is a sensitive and specific ancillary tool for diagnosing secretory carcinoma of the salivary gland and detecting ETV6–NTRK3 fusion. Histopathology 2020;76(3):375–82.
4. Klubíčková N, Kinkor Z, Michal M, et al. Epithelioid Soft Tissue Neoplasm of the Soft Palate with a PTCH1-GLI1 Fusion: A Case Report and Review of the Literature. Head Neck Pathol 2022;16(2):621–30.
5. Palsgrove DN, Rooper LM, Stevens TM, et al. GLI1-Altered Soft Tissue Tumors of the Head and Neck: Frequent Oropharyngeal Involvement, p16 Immunoreactivity, and Detectable Alterations by DDIT3 Break Apart FISH. Head Neck Pathol 2022;16(4):1146–56.
6. Liu YJ, Wagner MJ, Kim EY, et al. TUBA1A-GLI1 fusion in a soft tissue myoepithelial neoplasm. Hum Pathol Case Rep 2021;24:200497.
7. Lopez-Nunez O, Surrey LF, Alaggio R, et al. Novel APOD-GLI1 rearrangement in a sarcoma of unknown lineage. Histopathology 2021;78(2):338–40.

8. Nitta Y, Takeda M, Fujii T, et al. A case of pericytic neoplasm in the shoulder with a novel DERA-GLI1 gene fusion. Histopathology 2021;78(3):466–9.

9. Kerr DA, Pinto A, Subhawong TK, et al. Pericytoma With t(7;12) and ACTB-GLI1 Fusion: Reevaluation of an Unusual Entity and its Relationship to the Spectrum of GLI1 Fusion-related Neoplasms. Am J Surg Pathol 2019;43(12):1682–92.

10. Bridge JA, Sanders K, Huang D, et al. Pericytoma with t(7;12) and ACTB-GLI1 fusion arising in bone. Hum Pathol 2012;43(9):1524–9.

11. Castro E, Cortes-Santiago N, Ferguson LMS, et al. Translocation t(7;12) as the sole chromosomal abnormality resulting in ACTB-GLI1 fusion in pediatric gastric pericytoma. Hum Pathol 2016;53:137–41.

12. Prall OWJ, McEvoy CRE, Byrne DJ, et al. A Malignant Neoplasm From the Jejunum With a MALAT1-GLI1 Fusion and 26-Year Survival History. Int J Surg Pathol 2020;28(5):553–62.

13. Pettus JR, Kerr DA, Stan RV, et al. Primary myxoid and epithelioid mesenchymal tumor of the kidney with a novel GLI1-FOXO4 fusion. Genes Chromosomes Cancer 2021;60(2):116–22.

14. Argani P, Boyraz B, Oliva E, et al. GLI1 Gene Alterations in Neoplasms of the Genitourinary and Gynecologic Tract. Am J Surg Pathol 2022;46(5):677–87.

15. Koh NWC, Seow WY, Lee YT, et al. Pericytoma With t(7;12): The First Ovarian Case Reported and a Review of the Literature. Int J Gynecol 2019;38(5):479–84.

16. Punjabi LS, Goh CHR, Sittampalam K. Expanding the spectrum of GLI1-altered mesenchymal tumors-A high-grade uterine sarcoma harboring a novel PAMR1::GLI1 fusion and literature review of GLI1-altered mesenchymal neoplasms of the gynecologic tract. Genes Chromosomes Cancer 2023; 62(2):107–14.

17. Hui L, Bai Q, Yang W, et al. GLI1-rearranged mesenchymal tumor in the ovary. Histopathology 2022; 81(5):688–92. https://doi.org/10.1111/his.14785.

18. Ichikawa D, Yamashita K, Okuno Y, et al. Integrated diagnosis based on transcriptome analysis in suspected pediatric sarcomas. NPJ Genomic Med 2021;6:49.

19. Spans L, Fletcher CD, Antonescu CR, et al. Recurrent MALAT1-GLI1 oncogenic fusion and GLI1 upregulation define a subset of plexiform fibromyxoma. J Pathol 2016;239(3):335–43.

20. Graham RP, Nair AA, Davila JI, et al. Gastroblastoma harbors a recurrent somatic MALAT1-GLI1 fusion gene. Mod Pathol 2017;30(10):1443–52.

21. Agaram NP, Zhang L, Sung YS, et al. GLI1-amplifications expand the spectrum of soft tissue neoplasms defined by GLI1 gene fusions. Mod PatholInc 2019;32(11):1617–26.

22. Xu B, Chang K, Folpe AL, et al. Head and Neck Mesenchymal Neoplasms With GLI1 Gene Alterations: A Pathologic Entity With Distinct Histologic Features and Potential for Distant Metastasis. Am J Surg Pathol 2020;44(6):729–37.

23. Liu J, Mao R, Lao IW, et al. GLI1-altered mesenchymal tumor: a clinicopathological and molecular analysis of ten additional cases of an emerging entity. Virchows Arch Int J Pathol 2022;480(5):1087–99.

24. Dickson BC, Bishop JA. GLI1-altered soft tissue tumour. In: WHO Classification of Tumours Editorial Board. Head and Neck Tumours. vol. 9. 5th edition. WHO classification of tumours series. International Agency for Research on Cancer. 2022.

25. Rodrigues Simoes NJ, Tse JY, Faquin W, et al. Mesenchymal Neoplasms With ACTB-GLI1 Fusion: Towards a Better Understanding of This Enigmatic and Evolving Tumor Type (abs#65). In USCAP 2022 Abstracts: Bone and Soft Tissue Pathology (24-73). Mod Pathol 2022;35(2):63.

26. Aivazian K, Mahar A, Jackett LA, et al. GLI activated epithelioid cell tumour: report of a case and proposed new terminology. Pathology 2021;53(2):267–70.

27. Papke DJ, Dickson BC, Oliveira AM, et al. Distinctive Nested Glomoid Neoplasm: Clinicopathologic Analysis of 20 Cases of a Mesenchymal Neoplasm With Frequent GLI1 Alterations and Indolent Behavior. Am J Surg Pathol 2023;47(1):12–24.

28. Shahabi A, Israel AK, Sullivan CB, et al. Fine needle aspiration biopsy of epithelioid-mesenchymal neoplasm with PTCH1-GLI1 fusion: A case report. Diagn Cytopathol 2022;50(8):E223–9.

29. Zhong H, Xu C, Chen X, et al. GLI1-altered epithelioid soft tissue tumor: A newly described entity with a predilection for the tongue. Oral Surg Oral Med Oral Pathol Oral Radiol 2022;134(1):e14–22.

30. Jessurun J, Orr C, McNulty SN, et al. GLI1 -Rearranged Enteric Tumor : Expanding the Spectrum of Gastrointestinal Neoplasms With GLI1 Gene Fusions. Am J Surg Pathol 2023;47(1):65–73.

31. Zeng Y, Yao H, Jiang X, et al. GLI1-altered Mesenchymal Tumor Involving the Duodenum: Case Report and Literature Review. Int J Surg Pathol 2023. https://doi.org/10.1177/10668969231157782, 10668969231157782.

32. Alwaqfi RR, Samuelson MI, Guseva NN, et al. PTCH1-GLI1 Fusion-Positive Ovarian Tumor: Report of a Unique Case With Response to Tyrosine Kinase Inhibitor Pazopanib. J Natl Compr Cancer Netw JNCCN 2021;19(9):998–1004.

33. Machado I, Hosler GA, Traves V, et al. Superficial GLI1-amplified mesenchymal neoplasms: Expanding the spectrum of an emerging entity which reaches the realm of dermatopathology. J Cutan Pathol 2022;50(6):487–99.

34. Rollins BT, Cassarino DS, Lindberg M. Primary cutaneous epithelioid mesenchymal neoplasm with ACTB-GLI1 fusion: a case report. J Cutan Pathol 2022;49(3):284–7.

35. Parrack PH, Mariño-Enríquez A, Fletcher CDM, et al. GLI1 Immunohistochemistry Distinguishes Mesenchymal Neoplasms With GLI1 Alterations From Morphologic Mimics. Am J Surg Pathol 2023;47(4):453–60.

36. Hung YP, Fletcher CDM. Myopericytomatosis: Clinicopathologic Analysis of 11 Cases With Molecular Identification of Recurrent PDGFRB Alterations in Myopericytomatosis and Myopericytoma. Am J Surg Pathol 2017;41(8):1034–44.

37. Iwamura R, Komatsu K, Kusano M, et al. PDGFRB and NOTCH3 Mutations are Detectable in a Wider Range of Pericytic Tumors, Including Myopericytomas, Angioleiomyomas, Glomus Tumors, and Their Combined Tumors. Mod Pathol Off J U S Can Acad Pathol Inc 2023;36(3):100070.

38. Papke DJ, Dickson BC, Sholl L, et al. Pseudoendocrine Sarcoma: Clinicopathologic Analysis of 23 Cases of a Distinctive Soft Tissue Neoplasm With Metastatic Potential, Recurrent CTNNB1 Mutations, and a Predilection for Truncal Locations. Am J Surg Pathol 2022;46(1):33–43.

39. Kinzler KW, Bigner SH, Bigner DD, et al. Identification of an amplified, highly expressed gene in a human glioma. Science 1987;236(4797):70–3.

40. Rao SK, Edwards J, Joshi AD, et al. A survey of glioblastoma genomic amplifications and deletions. J Neuro Oncol 2010;96(2):169–79.

41. Roberts WM, Douglass EC, Peiper SC, et al. Amplification of the gli gene in childhood sarcomas. Cancer Res 1989;49(19):5407–13.

42. Gordon AT, Brinkschmidt C, Anderson J, et al. A novel and consistent amplicon at 13q31 associated with alveolar rhabdomyosarcoma. Genes Chromosomes Cancer 2000;28(2):220–6.

43. Simon R, Struckmann K, Schraml P, et al. Amplification pattern of 12q13-q15 genes (MDM2, CDK4, GLI) in urinary bladder cancer. Oncogene 2002; 21(16):2476–83.

Myxoid Pleomorphic Liposarcoma

Josephine K. Dermawan, MD, PhD

KEYWORDS

- Myxoid pleomorphic liposarcoma • TP53 • Loss of heterozygosity

---

Key points

- Myxoid pleomorphic liposarcoma (MPLPS) shows a strong predilection for the mediastinum and is a clinically aggressive sarcoma.
- Histologically, MPLPS is characterized by hybrid morphologic features of myxoid/round cell liposarcoma (MRLPS) and pleomorphic liposarcoma (PLPS).
- The most consistent molecular feature of MPLPS is recurrent *TP53* mutations and genome-wide loss of heterozygosity.

ABSTRACT

Myxoid pleomorphic liposarcoma (MPLPS) shows a strong predilection for the mediastinum and can affect a wide age range. Clinically, MPLPS exhibits aggressive behavior and demonstrates a worse overall and progression-free survival than myxoid/round cell liposarcoma (MRLPS) and pleomorphic liposarcoma (PLPS). Histologically, MPLPS is characterized by hybrid morphologic features of MRLPS and PLPS, including myxoid stroma, chicken wire-like vasculature, univacuolated and multivacuolated lipoblasts, and high-grade pleomorphic sarcomatous components. In terms of molecular features, MPLPS is distinct from other lipomatous tumors as it harbors genome-wide loss of heterozygosity.

INTRODUCTION

As early as the late 80s and 90s, oncologists and pathologists have observed a subset of liposarcomas that seem to show a predilection for the mediastinum and a tendency to affect younger adults.[1,2] This group of liposarcomas was thought to encompass a mixture of lipomatous tumors, such as well-differentiated/de-differentiated liposarcomas (WDLPS/DDLPS) with myxoid changes, myxoid/round cell liposarcoma (MRLPS), and pleomorphic liposarcoma (PLPS).[3,4] However, increasingly it was recognized that there may be a distinct liposarcomatous entity with the aforementioned clinical features that does not fit neatly into well-established categories.[5] For example, although WDLPS/DDLPS may also involve the mediastinum, it primarily affects older adults. MRLPS, like most other soft tissue tumors with a recurrent genetic alteration (*FUS/EWSR1::DDIT3*), contains monotonous ovoid-to-plump spindle cells and occasional signet-ring like lipoblasts, and should not demonstrate significant nuclear pleomorphism. Eventually, the term "myxoid pleomorphic liposarcoma" (MPLPS) was coined to describe this group of liposarcomas that predominantly occurs in the mediastinum of younger adults, demonstrating morphologic features shared by MRLPS and PLPS.[5] Although rare, a recent case series has also shown that MPLPS can affect patients of a broader age range than previously thought, including children and older adults.[6]

RADIOGRAPHIC FEATURES

On imaging studies, such as computed tomography of the chest, MPLPS often manifests as a large, heterogeneously enhancing soft tissue mass in the mediastinum that compresses and invades surrounding anatomic organs and structures, such as the pleura, lungs, chest wall, and pericardium (**Fig. 1**A). On magnetic resonance imaging, MPLPS can demonstrate fat attenuation signals internally.[6]

Robert J. Tomsich Pathology and Laboratory Medicine Institute, Cleveland Clinic, 9500 Euclid Avenue L25, Cleveland, OH 44195, USA
E-mail address: dermawj@ccf.org

Surgical Pathology 17 (2024) 25–29
https://doi.org/10.1016/j.path.2023.06.005
1875-9181/24/© 2023 Elsevier Inc. All rights reserved.

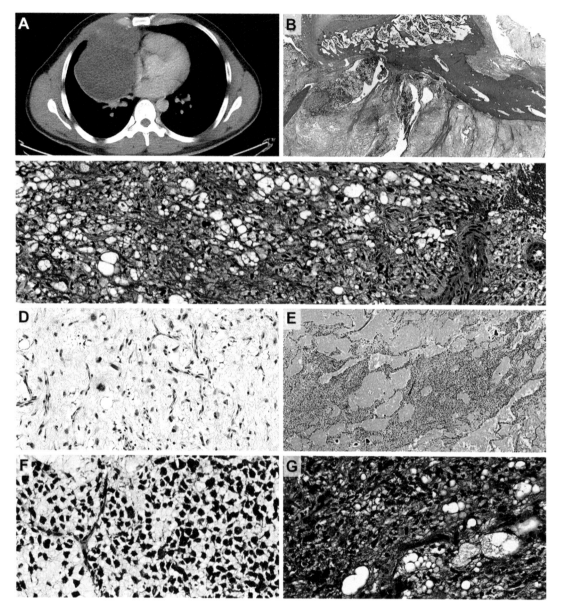

Fig. 1. (*A*), Computed tomography (CT) chest (transverse section) demonstrating a large right-sided mediastinal soft tissue mass compressing surrounding viscera, including the right lung and pericardium. (*B*), Low-power view of a case of MPLPS with myxoid stroma broadly infiltrating surrounding lamellar bone from the rib cage. (*C*), Intermediate magnification demonstrating admixture of chicken wire-like vasculature, uni- and multi-vacuolated lipoblasts, and ovoid plump spindle cells set in myxoid stroma. (*D*), Myxoid liposarcoma (MLPS)-like, relatively paucicellular areas with delicate, thin-walled plexiform vasculature and scattered lipoblasts. (*E*), "Pulmonary edema"-like areas with mucin pools, reminiscent of MLPS. (*F*), Round cell liposarcoma-like areas showing spindle to round cells with enlarged, hyperchromatic nuclei. (*G*), High-grade, pleomorphic liposarcoma-like, hypercellular areas containing multivacuolated pleomorphic lipoblasts and spindle cells with severe nuclear atypia.

GROSS FEATURES

Macroscopically, MPLPS appears as a large mass with a heterogeneously gelatinous-to-solid, yellow cut surface. Often adherent to adjacent anatomic structures in the mediastinum, such as the chest wall, pleura, and pericardium, clean surgical margins are difficult to achieve, contributing to a high local recurrence rate.

MICROSCOPIC FEATURES

On low power, the tumor demonstrates an infiltrative margin invading surrounding structures, such as bone and fibromuscular tissue in the chest wall (**Fig. 1**B). Histopathologically, the hallmark of MPLPS is the presence of hybrid morphologic features characteristic of both MRLPS and PLPS (**Fig. 1**C).[5–7] Some areas demonstrate typical features of myxoid liposarcoma (MLPS): myxoid and lipomatous areas with plexiform or "chicken wire"-like vasculature admixed with relatively monomorphic, ovoid spindle cells with scant cytoplasm and univacuolated lipoblasts (**Fig. 1**D). Some cases also demonstrate "pulmonary edema"-like areas, where mucin pools are separated by thin vascular septa (**Fig. 1**E). Moreover, these areas with relatively low cellularity may transition to more cellular areas comprised of cells with enlarged, hyperchromatic nuclei, reminiscent of high-grade MLPS (round cell liposarcoma) (**Fig. 1**F). However, often intimately admixed with these more uniform spindle cells and signet ring-like lipoblasts are multivacuolated, pleomorphic lipoblasts and spindle cells with increased nuclear pleomorphism and atypia, exceeding what is typically seen in MRLPS and more characteristic of PLPS (**Fig. 1**G). Additionally, these lipomatous areas can transition, sometimes abruptly, to high-grade non-lipomatous sarcomatous components that resemble undifferentiated pleomorphic sarcoma with significant degree of anaplasia.

MOLECULAR PATHOLOGY FEATURES

The most consistent and reproducible genetic alterations in MPLPS are the presence of *TP53* point mutations, most of which are either hotspot missense mutations or loss-of-function mutations (eg, truncating or splice site mutations), as well as genome-wide loss of heterozygosity (LOH) (**Fig. 2**A).[6,8] Other reported mutations, such as *RB1* deletion or inactivating mutations, do not appear to be as reproducible across all cases, observed in 25-67% of reported cases.[6,7] Widespread LOH is not observed in MRLPS or PLPS (**Fig. 2**B).[6] Genome-wide LOH may be detected by using array comparative genomic hybridization (array CGH)[8] or a comprehensive targeted DNA next-generation sequencing panel that includes the ability to interrogate allele-specific copy number profiles in its bioinformatics pipeline, using an analysis tool such as FACETS.[9] Since greater than 80% of the genome is involved by LOH, MPLPS may appear to show a haploid genome, similar to inflammatory rhabdomyoblastic tumor (IRMT) (formerly known as inflammatory leiomyosarcoma or histiocyte-rich rhabdomyoblastic tumor).[10–13] Interestingly, when MPLPS metastasizes or progresses, it can undergo whole genome doubling and show a pseudo-diploid karyotype, similar to the phenomenon observed when IRMT

progresses to rhabdomyosarcoma.[6,14] Copy number profiling will also demonstrate nonrecurrent chromosomal arm level amplifications and deletions.[6,7,15] Methylation profiling does not appear to be particularly helpful: at least one study reported that PLPS and MPLPS showed similar methylation profile on unsupervised clustering analysis.[7]

DIFFERENTIAL DIAGNOSIS

The differential diagnosis of MPLPS largely consists of other malignant lipomatous tumors, including PLPS, WDLPS/DDLPS, and MRLPS. Since a significant percentage of PLPS also harbor *TP53* mutations,[16] the presence of widespread LOH is a genomic feature that helps distinguish MPLPS from PLPS, which could be challenging on a morphologic basis alone, particularly if outside the mediastinum, as myxoid change (especially myxofibrosarcoma-like morphology) in PLPS is a well-known phenomenon.[17,18] Further, to rule out DDLPS with homologous lipoblastic differentiation or the myxoid variant of DDLPS,[19,20] the presence of *MDM2/CDK4* amplification must be excluded prior to rendering a diagnosis of MPLPS.[21] Likewise, the absence of *DDIT3* rearrangement should be established to exclude MRLPS.[22]

DIAGNOSIS

The diagnosis of MPLPS should be entertained in the setting of a large lipomatous tumor in the mediastinum of younger adults. Usually in such a clinical context, the presence of hybrid histologic features of MRLPS and PLPS is sufficient to support a diagnosis of MPLPS. This distinction is important given the worse prognosis of MPLPS compared to other lipomatous tumors that could enter its differential diagnosis (see later in discussion). However, in the absence of one or more of these hallmark clinicopathologic features, ancillary molecular studies demonstrating widespread LOH and *TP53* mutations, and the absence of genetic alterations characteristic of other lipomatous tumors, could help confirm or rule out MPLPS.

PROGNOSIS

The prognosis of MPLPS is poor. MPLPS has a high local recurrence rate and can also metastasize to distal sites. Compared to both MLPS (including high-grade MLPS) and PLPS, MPLPS has a significantly lower progression-free and overall survival rate. The high recurrence rate is likely due to difficulties in achieving disease-free margins and the involvement of vital anatomic organs in the mediastinum.[6]

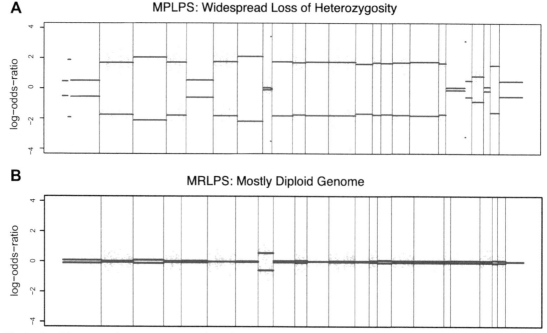

Fig. 2. Graphic output from FACETS, an algorithm designed to measure allele-specific copy number alterations, demonstrating genome-wide loss of heterozygosity (LOH) in a case of myxoid pleomorphic liposarcoma (*A*), as shown by the log odds ratio (log OR), a measurement of LOH based on the distribution of single nucleotide polymorphisms in the minor and total alleles.[9] In contrast, a case of myxoid/round cell liposarcoma demonstrates little to no LOH (*B*).

SUMMARY

MPLPS is a distinct lipomatous tumor clinically characterized by a strong predilection for the mediastinum in younger adults, but could affect a broad age range, and is associated with an aggressive clinical course, with frequent local recurrence and distant metastasis. The hallmark histologic finding is the presence of hybrid features characteristically seen in MRLPS and PLPS. On molecular profiling, MPLPS harbors recurrent *TP53* mutations. The defining genetic feature of MPLPS is genome wide LOH.

CLINICS CARE POINTS

- Clinically aggressive malignancy with predilection for the mediastinum of young adults.

- Lipomatous tumor with admixture of morphologic features of myxoid liposarcoma and pleomorphic liposarcoma.

- Allele-specific copy number profiling demonstrates widespread loss of heterozygosity.

- Negative for *MDM2* amplification and *FUS/EWSR1::DDIT3* fusions.

DISCLOSURE

The author has nothing to disclose.

REFERENCES

1. Plukker JT, Joosten HJ, Rensing JB, et al. Primary liposarcoma of the mediastinum in a child. J Surg Oncol 1988;37(4):257–63.
2. Greif J, Marmor S, Merimsky O, et al. Primary liposarcoma of the mediastinum. Sarcoma 1998; 2(3–4):205–7.
3. Hahn HP, Fletcher CDM. Primary mediastinal liposarcoma: clinicopathologic analysis of 24 cases. Am J Surg Pathol 2007;31(12):1868–74.
4. Boland JM, Colby TV, Folpe AL. Liposarcomas of the mediastinum and thorax: a clinicopathologic and molecular cytogenetic study of 24 cases, emphasizing unusual and diverse histologic features. Am J Surg Pathol 2012;36(9):1395–403.
5. Alaggio R, Coffin CM, Weiss SW, et al. Liposarcomas in young patients: a study of 82 cases occurring in patients younger than 22 years of age. Am J Surg Pathol 2009;33(5):645–58.
6. Dermawan JK, Hwang S, Wexler L, et al. Myxoid pleomorphic liposarcoma is distinguished from other liposarcomas by widespread loss of heterozygosity and significantly worse overall survival: a genomic and clinicopathologic study. Mod Pathol 2022;35(11):1644–55.

7. Creytens D, Folpe AL, Koelsche C, et al. Myxoid pleomorphic liposarcoma-a clinicopathologic, immunohistochemical, molecular genetic and epigenetic study of 12 cases, suggesting a possible relationship with conventional pleomorphic liposarcoma. Mod Pathol 2021;34(11):2043–9.

8. Hofvander J, Jo VY, Ghanei I, et al. Comprehensive genetic analysis of a paediatric pleomorphic myxoid liposarcoma reveals near-haploidization and loss of the RB1 gene. Histopathology 2016;69(1):141–7.

9. Shen R, Seshan VE. FACETS: allele-specific copy number and clonal heterogeneity analysis tool for high-throughput DNA sequencing. Nucleic Acids Res 2016;44(16):e131.

10. Dal Cin P, Sciot R, Fletcher CD, et al. Inflammatory leiomyosarcoma may be characterized by specific near-haploid chromosome changes. J Pathol 1998;185(1):112–5.

11. Arbajian E, Köster J, Vult von Steyern F, et al. Inflammatory leiomyosarcoma is a distinct tumor characterized by near-haploidization, few somatic mutations, and a primitive myogenic gene expression signature. Mod Pathol 2018;31(1):93–100.

12. Martinez AP, Fritchie KJ, Weiss SW, et al. Histiocyte-rich rhabdomyoblastic tumor: rhabdomyosarcoma, rhabdomyoma, or rhabdomyoblastic tumor of uncertain malignant potential? A histologically distinctive rhabdomyoblastic tumor in search of a place in the classification of skeletal muscle neoplasms. Mod Pathol 2019;32(3):446–57.

13. Cloutier JM, Charville GW, Mertens F, et al. Inflammatory Leiomyosarcoma" and "Histiocyte-rich Rhabdomyoblastic Tumor": a clinicopathological, immunohistochemical and genetic study of 13 cases, with a proposal for reclassification as "Inflammatory Rhabdomyoblastic Tumor. Mod Pathol 2021;34(4):758–69.

14. Geiersbach K, Kleven DT, Blankenship HT, et al. Inflammatory rhabdomyoblastic tumor with progression to high-grade rhabdomyosarcoma. Mod Pathol 2021;34(5):1035–6.

15. Creytens D, van Gorp J, Ferdinande L, et al. Array-based comparative genomic hybridization analysis of a pleomorphic myxoid liposarcoma. J Clin Pathol 2014;67(9):834–5.

16. Barretina J, Taylor BS, Banerji S, et al. Subtype-specific genomic alterations define new targets for soft-tissue sarcoma therapy. Nat Genet 2010;42(8):715–21.

17. Hornick JL, Bosenberg MW, Mentzel T, et al. Pleomorphic liposarcoma: clinicopathologic analysis of 57 cases. Am J Surg Pathol 2004;28(10):1257–67.

18. Gjorgova Gjeorgjievski S, Thway K, Dermawan JK, et al. Pleomorphic Liposarcoma: A Series of 120 Cases With Emphasis on Morphologic Variants. Am J Surg Pathol 2022;46(12):1700–5.

19. Mariño-Enríquez A, Fletcher CDM, Dal Cin P, et al. Dedifferentiated liposarcoma with "homologous" lipoblastic (pleomorphic liposarcoma-like) differentiation: clinicopathologic and molecular analysis of a series suggesting revised diagnostic criteria. Am J Surg Pathol 2010;34(8):1122–31.

20. Hisaoka M, Morimitsu Y, Hashimoto H, et al. Retroperitoneal liposarcoma with combined well-differentiated and myxoid malignant fibrous histiocytoma-like myxoid areas. Am J Surg Pathol 1999;23(12):1480–92.

21. Weaver J, Downs-Kelly E, Goldblum JR, et al. Fluorescence in situ hybridization for MDM2 gene amplification as a diagnostic tool in lipomatous neoplasms. Mod Pathol 2008;21(8):943–9.

22. Rabbitts TH, Forster A, Larson R, et al. Fusion of the dominant negative transcription regulator CHOP with a novel gene FUS by translocation t(12;16) in malignant liposarcoma. Nat Genet 1993;4(2):175–80.

Sarcomas with *EWSR1::Non-ETS* Fusion (*EWSR1::NFATC2* and *EWSR1::PATZ1*)

Isidro Machado, MD, PhD[a,b,c,1,*],
Antonio Llombart-Bosch, MD, PhD[d],
Gregory W. Charville, MD, PhD[e], Samuel Navarro, MD, PhD[d],
María Purificación Domínguez Franjo, MD PhD[f],
Julia A. Bridge, MD[g,h], Konstantinos Linos, MD[i,1,*]

KEYWORDS

- *EWSR1::non-ETS* sarcoma • *EWSR1::NFATC2* sarcoma • *EWSR1::PATZ1* sarcoma
- Undifferentiated round cell sarcoma

Key points

- *EWSR1/FUS::NFATC2* and *EWSR1::PATZ1* sarcomas are a novel molecular subset of undifferentiated round cell sarcomas of bone and soft tissue with particular clinical and histomorphologic features. Interpretation of any molecular findings requires thorough clinical-morphologic correlation.

- *EWSR1/FUS::NFATC2* sarcomas in adult patients occur more commonly in bone than in soft tissue and consist of tumor cells arranged in anastomosing cords/clusters and cribriform/pseudoacinar structures embedded within abundant myxohyaline, sclerotic, or chondromyxoid matrix.

- A combination of CD99, PAX7, NKX2.2, NKX3.1, and AGGRECAN immunostaining may detect most *EWSR1/FUS::NFATC2* sarcomas. Fluorescence in situ hybridization (FISH) using *EWSR1* and *FUS* break-apart probes and/or *EWSR1::NFATC2* and *FUS::NFATC2* fusion probes are useful for the detection of *EWSR1* or *FUS* rearrangement, fusion, and amplification.

ABSTRACT

The wide application of increasingly advanced molecular studies in routine clinical practice has allowed a detailed, albeit still incomplete, genetic subclassification of undifferentiated round cell sarcomas. The WHO classification continues to include provisional molecular entities, whose clinicopathologic features are in the early stages of evolution. This review focuses on the clinicopathologic, molecular, and prognostic features of undifferentiated round cell sarcomas with *EWSR1/FUS::NFATC2* or *EWSR1::PATZ1* fusions. Classic histopathologic findings, uncommon variations, and diagnostic pitfalls are addressed, along with the utility of recently developed immunohistochemical and molecular markers.

[a] Pathology Department, Instituto Valenciano de Oncología, Valencia, Spain; [b] Patologika Laboratory, Hospital Quiron-Salud, Valencia, Spain; [c] Pathology Department, University of Valencia, Valencia, Spain; [d] Pathology Department, university of Valencia, Spain and Cancer CIBER (CIBERONC), Madrid, Spain; [e] Department of Pathology, Stanford University, Stanford, CA, USA; [f] Pathology Department, Hospital Ruber Internacional, Madrid, Spain; [g] Department of Pathology and Microbiology, University of Nebraska Medical Center, Omaha, NE, USA; [h] Division of Molecular Pathology, ProPath, Dallas, TX, USA; [i] Department of Pathology & Laboratory Medicine, Memorial Sloan Kettering Cancer Center, New York, NY, USA
[1] Both authors have equally contributed.
* Corresponding authors. Department of Pathology & Laboratory Medicine, Memorial Sloan Kettering Cancer Center, New York, NY, USA
E-mail addresses: Isidro.machado@uv.es (I.M.); linosk@mskcc.org (K.L.)

Surgical Pathology 17 (2024) 31–55
https://doi.org/10.1016/j.path.2023.07.001
1875-9181/24/© 2023 Elsevier Inc. All rights reserved.

- *EWSR1::PATZ1* sarcomas arise in deep soft tissue and show a predilection for the chest wall and abdomen. They may show variably thick sclerotic bands forming multiple lobules, hyalinized or myxohyaline stromal tissue and can exhibit low- to overtly high-grade spindle or round cell morphology.

- Almost all *EWSR1::PATZ1* sarcomas show coexpression of neural and myogenic markers; CD99 immunoreactivity is occasional. Because of the close proximity of *EWSR1* and *PATZ1* on 22q12.2, molecular approaches, such as reverse transcription polymerase chain reaction or RNA sequencing, are preferable over FISH. The detection of the specific gene fusion is essential for a definitive diagnosis.

OVERVIEW

The detection of a well-described oncogenic fusion is an important clinical tool in sarcomas, as clinical behavior and tumor biology are significantly impacted by the fusion driver.[1–9] However, with the increasing detection of driver gene fusions, their specificity has inevitably been reduced.[3–19] *EWSR1* is a classic example of a gene's promiscuity in the biology of mesenchymal tumors; it is detected in a continuously expanding list of various benign and malignant tumors with distinct morphologic and clinical characteristics.[1–19] Ewing sarcoma (ES) represents the prototypical entity of undifferentiated round cell sarcoma. It harbors *EWSR1* or much rarer *FUS*

rearrangements with any of the *ETS* genes (*FLI1*, *ERG*, *ETV4*, *FEV*).[1–4,6–18] *EWSR1::FLI1* is the most frequent fusion (~85%), whereas *EWSR1::ERG* is the second most common (~10%).[1–4,6–18]

With the advent of next-generation sequencing (NGS) technology, novel molecular subsets of undifferentiated round cell sarcomas have emerged; some of them are well-characterized (eg, *CIC*-rearranged and *BCOR*-altered sarcomas), whereas those with *EWSR1/FUS::non-ETS* fusions are significantly less frequent.[5–34] This last subgroup includes sarcomas with *EWSR1/FUS::NFATC2* and *EWSR1::PATZ1* fusions, which are epigenetically distinct from classic ES according to DNA methylation-based classification.[13,24–26,35–64] To

Table 1
EWSR1::NFATC2

Case	Study	Age/Gender	Location	Histopathology	IHC positive	IHC negative	Outcome	Follow-up months
1	Ishida et al, 1992	26/F	Femur	Small round cell, nests, cord and trabeculae. Fibrous to myxohyaline stroma	NR	NR	NR	NR
2	Szuhai et al, 2009	39/M	Right humerus	Small round, epithelioid and clear cells, cords, solid pattern with minimal fibrous stromal tissue	CD99	Keratin, desmin, S100	NR	NR
3	Szuhai et al, 2009	16/M	Right femur	Small round cells, cords, solid pattern with fibrous stromal tissue	CD99	Keratin, desmin, S100	NR	NR
4	Szuhai et al, 2009	21/M	Right thigh	Small round, epithelioid, clear cells, nested pattern with moderate sclerotic stroma	CD99 patchy	Keratin, desmin, S100	NR	NR
5	Szuhai et al, 2009	25/M	Right femur	Small round cells, cords, solid pattern with fibrous stromal tissue	CD99	Keratin, desmin, S100	NR	NR
6	Wang et al, 2012	NR	NR	NR	NR	NR	NR	NR
7	Romeo et al, 2012	32/M	Lower extremity bone	Pleomorphic epithelioid clear cells, solid pattern with scarce stroma	CD99, EMA, keratin (DL), calponin	S100, p63, GFAP	NED	64
8	Sadri et al, 2014	30/M	Left femur	Epithelioid, clear cells, nests, solid pattern, abundant and fibrous stroma	CD99, keratin (DL)	EMA, desmin, S100, p63	LR	30
9	Kinkor et al, 2014	12/M	Left humerus	Epithelioid, clear cells, tumor nests with moderate fibrous stroma	CD99	EMA, keratin, S100, calponin, p63	NED	11
10	Kinkor et al, 2014	28/M	Left femur	Epithelioid, clear cells, tumor nests with moderate fibrous stroma	CD99	EMA, keratin, S100, calponin, p63	LR and lung Mtx	48
11	Brohl et al, 2014	15/M	Femur	NR	NR	NR	NR	NR
12	Cohen et al, 2018	24/F	Left calf	Small round cells tumor with cords, trabeculae with abundant fibromyxoid stroma	CD99 patchy, keratin (DL), EMA (DL)	Desmin, S100, calponin, p63, GFAP	NED	12
13-20	Baldauf et al, 2018	NR	NR	NR	NR	NR	NR	NR
21	Toki et al, 2018	NR	NR		NR	NR	NR	NR
22	Watson et al, 2018	32/M	Humerus	NR	NR	NR	NR	NR
23	Watson et al, 2018	12/F	Tibia	NR	NR	NR	NR	NR
24	Watson et al, 2018	61/M	Calf	NR	NR	NR	NR	NR
25	Watson et al, 2018	23/M	Femur	NR	NR	NR	NR	NR
26	Watson et al, 2018	33/M	Femur	NR	NR	NR	NR	NR
27	Watson et al, 2018	49/F	Femur	NR	NR	NR	NR	NR
28	Watson et al, 2018	43/M	Femur	NR	NR	NR	NR	NR
29	Yau et al, 2019	43/M	Femur	Small round cells tumor, solid pattern with minimal fibrous stromal tissue	CD99, keratin	NR	NED	12
30	Bode-Lesniewska et al, 2019	34/F	Femur	Small round cell tumor with trabeculae and fibrous stroma	CD99	Keratin, desmin, S100	Lung Mtx	132
31	Bode-Lesniewska et al,2019	42/M	Tibia	Small round cell tumor with trabeculae and nest. Fibrous stroma	CD99, EMA	Desmin, S100	NED	102
32	Bode-Lesniewska et al, 2019	60/F	Abdomen	Small round cell tumor with trabeculae and fibrous stroma	CD99, EMA (focal), keratin	Desmin, S100	NED	8
33	Bode-Lesniewska et al, 2019	12/M	Humerus	Spindle cell tumor with trabeculae and fibrous stroma.	CD99, EMA	Keratin, desmin, S100	NED	8

(continued on next page)

Table 1
(continued)

Case	Study	Age/Gender	Location	Histopathology	IHC positive	IHC negative	Outcome	Follow-up months
34	Wang et al, 2019	67/M	Left radius	Small round and/or epithelioid cells arranged in anastomosing cords. Abundant stroma myxoid/myxohyaline to collagenous	CD99, NKX2.2, EMA, AE1/AE3 (DL)	ERG, FLI1, desmin, SYN, chrom, S100, CCNB3, ETV4	NED	14
35	Wang et al, 2019	32/M	Periclavicular soft tissue	Small round and/or epithelioid cells arranged in anastomosing cords. Abundant stroma myxoid/myxohyaline to collagenous	CD99, NKX2.2, WT1, EMA	ERG, FLI1, desmin, SYN, chrom, S100, CCNB3, ETV4, AE1/AE3	NED	24
36	Wang et al, 2019	42/M	Right radius	Small round and/or epithelioid cells arranged in anastomosing cords. Abundant stroma myxoid/myxohyaline to collagenous	CD99, NKX2.2, WT1, EMA	ERG, FLI1, desmin, SYN, chrom, S100, CCNB3, ETV4, AE1/AE3	AWD	16
37	Wang et al, 2019	24/F	Gastrocnemius muscle	Small round and/or epithelioid cells arranged in anastomosing cords. Abundant stroma myxoid/myxohyaline to collagenous	CD99, NKX2.2, WT1, AE1/AE3 (DL)	ERG, FLI1, desmin, SYN, chrom, S100, CCNB3, ETV4	NED	23
38	Wang et al, 2019	42/M	Right radius	Solid pattern, matrix-poor areas, cells arranged in long parallel cords, necrosis	CD99, NKX2.2, EMA, AE1/AE3 (DL)	ERG, FLI1, desmin, SYN, chrom, S100, CCNB3, ETV4, EMA	DOD, bone and soft tissue Mtx	93
39	Wang et al, 2019	59/M	Left periclavicular soft tissue	Solid pattern, matrix-poor areas, cells arranged in long parallel cords, necrosis	CD99, NKX2.2, EMA	ERG, FLI1, desmin, SYN, chrom, S100, CCNB3, ETV4, AE1/AE3	LR, NED	144
40	Diaz-Perez et al, 2019	28/M	Tibia	Small round cells tumor, nests and cords with fibrous stromal tissue	CD99	EMA, keratin, desmin, S100	NED	8
41	Diaz-Perez et al, 2019	39/M	Femur	Epithelioid and spindle cell tumor, nests and cords with fibrous stromal tissue	CD99, EMA (focal)	Keratin, S100	NED	30
42	Diaz-Perez et al, 2019	28/M	Humerus	Epithelioid and spindle cell tumor, nests and cords with fibrous stromal tissue	CD99	Keratin, desmin, S100	NR	NR
43	Diaz-Perez et al, 2019	46/M	Femur	Epithelioid and spindle cell tumor, nests and cords and solid areas with fibrous stromal tissue	NR	CD99, EMA, keratin, desmin, S100	LR and lung Mtx	6
44	Koelsche et a, 2019	51/M	Humerus	Small round to polygonal with faint eosinophilic to clear cytoplasm, nested pattern and fibrous septae	NR	NR	NR	NR
45	Koelsche et a, 2019	39/M	Humerus	Small round to polygonal with faint eosinophilic to clear cytoplasm, nested pattern and fibrous septae	NR	NR	NR	NR
46	Koelsche et a, 2019	56/F	Femur	Small round to polygonal with faint eosinophilic to clear cytoplasm, nested pattern and fibrous septae	NR	NR	NR	NR
47	Koelsche et a, 2019	16/M	Femur	Small round to polygonal with faint eosinophilic to clear cytoplasm, nested pattern and fibrous septae	NR	NR	NR	NR
48	Koelsche et a, 2019	17/F	Humerus	Small round to polygonal with faint eosinophilic to clear cytoplasm, nested pattern and fibrous septae	NR	NR	NR	NR
49	Mantilla et al, 2019	67/M	Thigh/muscle	NR	NR	NR	NR	NR
50	Yoshida et al, 2020	39/M	Femur	Round/ovoid cell tumor with cord/nested/trabecular pattern and fibrotic, hyalinized, or myxoid background	NKX3.1	NR	NR	NR
51	Yoshida et al, 2020	46/M	Femur	Round/ovoid cell tumor with cord/nested/trabecular pattern and fibrotic, hyalinized, or myxoid background	NKX3.1	NR	NR	NR
52	Yoshida et al, 2020	27/M	Retroperitoneum	Round/ovoid cell tumor with cord/nested/trabecular pattern and fibrotic, hyalinized, or myxoid background	NKX3.1	NR	NR	NR
53	Yoshida et al, 2020	31/F	Scapula	Round/ovoid cell tumor with cord/nested/trabecular pattern and fibrotic, hyalinized, or myxoid background	NKX3.1	NR	NR	NR
54	Yoshida et al, 2020	36/M	Neck	Round/ovoid cell tumor with cord/nested/trabecular pattern and fibrotic, hyalinized, or myxoid background	NKX3.1	NR	NR	NR
55	Yoshida et al, 2020	51/M	Forearm	Round/ovoid cell tumor with cord/nested/trabecular pattern and fibrotic, hyalinized, or myxoid background	NKX3.1	NR	NR	NR
56	Yoshida et al, 2020	78/F	Tibia	Round/ovoid cell tumor	NKX3.1	NR	NR	NR
57	Yoshida et al, 2020	38/M	Thigh	Round/ovoid cell tumor with cord/nested/trabecular pattern and fibrotic, hyalinized, or myxoid background	NKX3.1	NR	NR	NR
58	Yoshida et al, 2020	44/M	Thigh	Round/ovoid cell tumor with cord/nested/trabecular pattern and fibrotic, hyalinized, or myxoid background	NKX3.1	NR	NR	NR
59	Yoshida et al, 2020, same case Machado et al, 2018	36F	Fibula	Round/ovoid cell tumor with cord/nested/trabecular pattern and fibrotic, hyalinized, or myxoid background. Abundant clear and epithelioid cells.	NKX3.1, CD99, NKX2.2, ETV4	NR	NR	NR
60	Yoshida et al, 2020	62/F	Femur	Round/ovoid cell tumor with cord/nested/trabecular pattern and fibrotic, hyalinized, or myxoid background	NKX3.1	NR	NR	NR
61	Yoshida et al, 2020	49/M	Tibia	Dense proliferation of uniform oval cells without a cord or nested pattern. Fascicular proliferation and anaplastic spindle cell post-chemotherapy.	NKX3.1	CD99, NKX2.2	DOD lung and brain Mtx	18

Case	Study	Age/Gender	Location	Histopathology	IHC positive	IHC negative	Outcome	Follow-up months
62	Perret et al, 2020	27/M	Tibia	Lobules and sheets of monotonous round/ovoid cells variably abundant fibrous to myxoid stroma. Low mitotic index.	CD99, AGG, NKX3.1 (F)	Keratin, desmin, S100, BCOR, ETV4, SATB2, ERG	NED	102
63	Perret et al, 2020	33/M	Femur	Lobules/sheets of monotonous round/ovoid cells with fibrous stroma and cartilaginous differentiation. High mitotic index.	CD99, AGG	Keratin, desmin, S100, BCOR, ETV4, SATB2, ERG, NKX3.1	DOD /Mtx	25
64	Perret et al, 2020	43/M	Femur	Lobules/sheets of monotonous round/ovoid cells with fibrous stroma and cartilaginous differentiation. High mitotic index.	CD99, AGG, WT1, NKX3.1 (F), keratin (F)	Desmin, S100, BCOR, ETV4, SATB2, ERG	DOD /Mtx	7
65	Perret et al, 2020	66/F	Femur	Lobules/sheets of monotonous round/ovoid cells with fibrous stroma. High mitotic index.	CD99, keratin, BCOR, ETV4, ERG, AGG	Desmin, S100, SATB2, NKX3.1	DOD/Mtx	32
66	Perret et al, 2020	28/F	Tibia	Lobules/sheets of monotonous round/ovoid cells with prominent collagen matrix .Low mitotic index.	CD99, AGG	Keratin, desmin, S100, SATB2, NKX3.2, ERG, ETV4, BCOR	NED	5
67	Perret et al, 2020	19/F	Ilium	Lobules/sheets of monotonous round/ovoid cells with fibrous stroma. Low mitotic index.	CD99, AGG	SATB2	AWD	8
68	Perret et al, 2020	58/M	Femur	Predominant spindle cells proliferation with cartilaginous differentiation. Low mitotic index.	CD99, keratin, AGG	Desmin, BCOR, NKX3.1	NR	NR
69	Tsuda et al, 2020	78/M	Tibia	Small round cell with fibrous stroma	NR	NR	NR	NR
70	Makise et al, 2021	26/F	Femur	Round /ovoid tumor cells arranged in nests or cords within a fibrous to myxohyaline background resembling an adamantinoma	NKX2.2, PAX7, NKX3.1	NR	AWD/ LR	24
71	Tsuchie et al. 2022	39/F	Soft tissue	NR	NR	NR	NR	NR
72	Shaheen et al. 2022	21/M	Tibia	Monomorphic round and epithelioid tumor with scattered spindle cells	CD99, NKX2.2, NKX3.1, SATB2, CK AE1/AE3	CK 34BE12, SS18-SSX, desmin, ERG, BCOR, S100, SOX10, MUC4, CD45, beta-catenin, GFAP, HMB45, MITF, Melan A, CD31	NED	8

Blue, *FUS::NFATC2* fusion, Red, soft tissue location.

Abbreviations: AGG, AGGRECAN; AWD, alive with disease; Chrom, Chromogranin-A; DL, Dot-like pattern; DOD, died of disease; GFAP, Glial Fibrillary Acidic Protein; LR, local recurrence; Mtx, metastasis; NED, no evidence of disease; NR, not reported; SYN, synaptophysin.

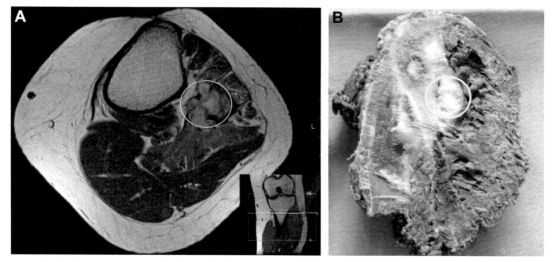

Fig. 1. MRI (*A*) and macroscopic findings (*B*) of an *EWSR1::NFATC2* sarcoma partially confined to the intramedullary cavity of the fibula with extension to the surrounding soft tissue (*Circle*). (Courtesy Dr. Antonina Parafioriti, Milan).

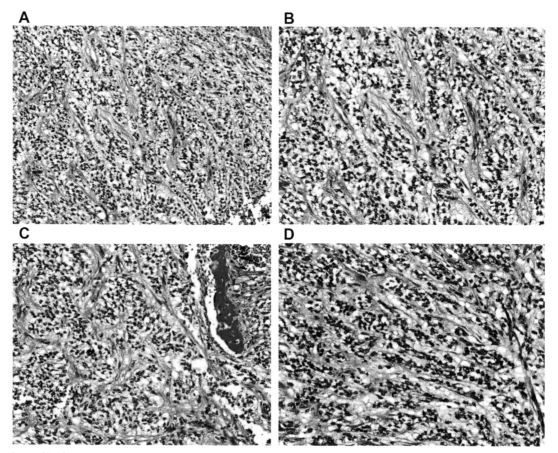

Fig. 2. (*A–C*) *EWSR1::NFATC2* sarcoma grows in lobules and sheets of round/oval to epithelioid cells with clear cytoplasm (hematoxylin and eosin [H&E], original magnification ×200 and ×400). (*D*) Cordlike pattern and chondromyxoid stromal tissue in an *EWSR1::NFATC2* sarcoma (H&E, original magnification ×600).

no surprise, these fusions have also been detected in unrelated neoplasms, another testament to the reduced specificity of these genetic events.[61–64] In particular, *EWSR1/FUS::NFATC2* has been detected in hemangiomas of bone and simple bone cysts,[61–64] whereas a subset of renal cell tumors (thyroid-like follicular carcinoma of the kidney), as well as primary central nervous system tumors, can harbor the *EWSR1::PATZ1* fusion.[65–70]

Because of the rarity of *EWSR1/FUS::non-ETS* fusions in undifferentiated round cell sarcomas, their clinical and histopathologic features are not well-defined.[35–70] In this review, the current understanding of undifferentiated round cell sarcomas with *EWSR1/FUS::NFATC2* and *EWSR1::PATZ1* fusions is summarized.

SARCOMAS WITH *EWSR1/FUS::NFATC2* FUSION TRANSCRIPT

Background

EWSR1::NFATC2 sarcoma was first described in 2009 by Szuhai and colleagues,[36] and since then, fewer than 100 cases have been documented (**Table 1**). This entity differs from ES with respect to its morphologic aspects, genomic/transcriptomic profile, and its limited response to neoadjuvant chemotherapy.[35–60] Seligson and colleagues[59] published the largest multiscale-omic study with data from 1024 *EWSR1*-rearranged sarcomas, in which 14 tumors with *EWSR1::NFATC2* fusion clustered separately from classic ES based on secondary genomic landscapes. Last, additional studies using methylome, transcriptome, and copy number analysis have shown convincing evidence that undifferentiated round cell sarcomas with *EWSR1/FUS::NFATC2* fusion represent an entity separate from conventional ES.[13,24–26]

Clinical and Radiologic Findings

EWSR1/FUS::NFATC2 sarcomas are rare neoplasms predominantly located in the bone, although tumors arising in the soft tissue have been sporadically reported[35–60] (see **Table 1**).

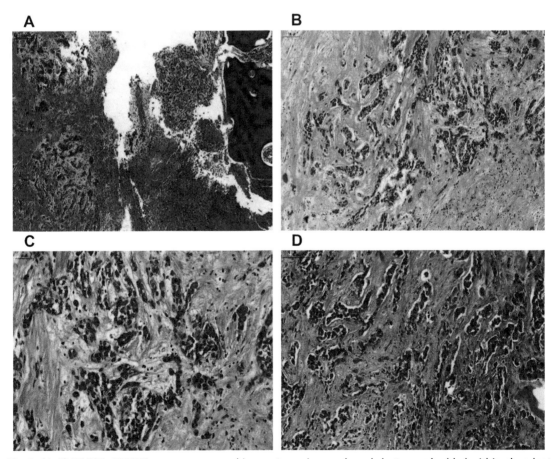

Fig. 3. (*A–D*) *EWSR1::NFATC2* sarcoma arranged in anastomosing cords and clusters embedded within abundant myxohyaline stroma (H&E, original magnification ×100, ×200, and ×400).

The metaphysis or diaphysis of long bones is the most frequent anatomic location, whereas soft tissue tumors can arise in the extremities, retroperitoneum, chest wall, and the head and neck area.[35–60] They display a strong male predominance, affecting young to middle-aged patients (see **Table 1**) with significant risk of local and distant recurrence, and poor response to ES-directed chemotherapy.

Radiologically, bone tumors (**Fig. 1A**) can occasionally be well-circumscribed, but usually exhibit a significant extracortical component with saucerization of the cortex associated with cortical buttressing.[41–53] Soft tissue tumors can also sometimes be well-circumscribed with a slow growth and long preoperative clinical history.[53]

Macroscopic Assessment and Histopathology Features

Macroscopically, *EWSR1/FUS::NFATC2* sarcomas have a wide size range and exhibit a yellowish-tan, firm or fleshy cut surface.[13,47–53] They are ill-defined and locally destructive and infiltrate into adjacent soft tissue, although occasionally they can be well-circumscribed or confined to the intramedullary cavity (see **Fig. 1B**).

Microscopically, *EWSR1/FUS/NFATC2* sarcomas are infiltrative at the periphery, growing in lobules and sheets.[13,45–59] They are typically monotonous, composed of round to oval or epithelioid cells, with variable nuclear hyperchromasia and eosinophilic or clear cytoplasm (**Figs. 2–5**). The mitotic activity can be brisk, and geographic necrosis can sometimes be encountered. The architecture is that of anastomosing cords, clusters, and cribriform/pseudoacinar structures embedded within variable myxohyaline, sclerotic/fibrous/collagenous, or chondromyxoid matrix, frequently resembling a myoepithelial tumor.[13,45–59] Rarely, they may display moderate nuclear pleomorphism, spindle cell growth pattern, or even neoplastic bone formation and/or cartilaginous differentiation.[51–53,55–58]

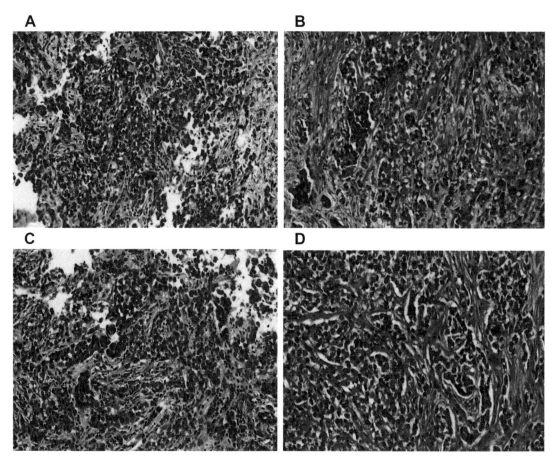

Fig. 4. (*A–D*) *EWSR1::NFATC2* sarcoma arranged in clusters and pseudoacinar structures with hyaline and fibrous stroma (H&E, original magnification ×200 and ×400).

Immunoprofile

By immunohistochemistry (**Fig. 6**), CD99 is almost always expressed (see **Fig. 6A–C**), and in approximately half of the cases, it shows diffuse immunoreactivity with membranous, cytoplasmic, and perinuclear dotlike patterns. NKX2.2 and PAX7 are also positive, whereas ETV4 expression is variable (see **Fig. 6**D).[13,46–58] Focal positivity for keratin AE1/AE3 (dotlike), EMA, and CD138 has been reported.[54–58] RNA expression profiling has identified differential NKX3.1 overexpression, which was later confirmed by RNA in situ hybridization and immunohistochemistry[54–56] (see **Fig. 6**E). Hence, NKX3.1 immunostain can be used diagnostically, as it is expressed in ~80% of *EWSR1::NFATC2* sarcomas,[54–56] whereas it is negative in many other round cell sarcomas, including ES, *CIC*-rearranged, and *BCOR*-genetically altered ones. A significant difference between *EWSR1::NFATC2* and *FUS::NFATC2* sarcomas is that NKX2.2, PAX7,

and NKX3.1 are not typically expressed in the latter; this is consistent with the differential downregulation of NKX3-1 in *FUS::NFATC2* sarcomas.[56] However, a recent study by Perret and colleagues[56] showed that AGGRECAN is a sensitive and specific marker for *NFATC2*-rearranged sarcomas, irrespective of the partner, as its expression in other round cell sarcomas is limited.

In summary, a combination of CD99, PAX7, NKX2.2, NKX3.1, and AGGRECAN will identify the great majority of *EWSR1/FUS::NFATC2* sarcomas.

Molecular Biology

EWSR1/FUS::NFATC2 sarcoma is likely the most common and phenotypically best-characterized tumor type among the category of round cell sarcomas with *EWSR1/FUS*::non-*ETS* fusions.[13,54–58] It is defined, most frequently, by the presence of a fusion between *EWSR1* (22q12.2) and *NFATC2*

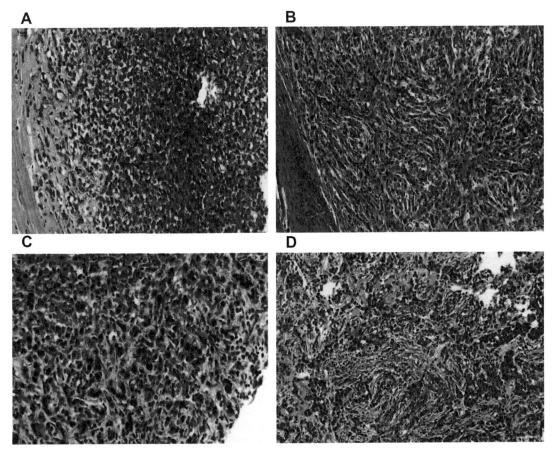

Fig. 5. *EWSR1::NFATC2* sarcoma with: (*A*) limited stromal tissue and diffuse solid sheets of tumor cells, closely resembling ES (H&E, original magnification ×400); (*B*) limited stromal tissue and diffuse solid sheets of ovoid/spindle cells, closely resembling *BCOR*-genetically altered sarcoma (H&E, original magnification ×400); (*C*) pleomorphic cells (H&E, original magnification ×400); (*D*) Pseudoacinar structures and cordlike arrangement resembling metastatic carcinoma (H&E, original magnification ×200).

(20q13.2),[13,54–58] often resulting from an unbalanced translocation and concomitant amplification (see **Figs. 6F and 7A**). In a small number of cases, an alternative, nonamplified *FUS::NFATC2* fusion is present.[13,56] Expression and methylome profiling have shown that undifferentiated round cell sarcomas with *EWSR1/FUS::NFATC2* cluster separately from ES, *EWSR1::PATZ1* sarcomas, *CIC*-rearranged and *BCOR*-genetically altered sarcomas, or myoepithelial tumors.[24–26,56]

NFATC2 is a member of the family of transcription factors responsible for T-cell differentiation and cytokine activation.[38–40] Genomic variants in *NFATC2* have been described in the pathogenesis of both solid and hematologic malignancies.[38–40] It is thought that dysregulation of NFATC2 is involved in multiple biological mechanisms of tumorigenesis, including the induction of tumor invasion, repression of tumor suppressor genes, and the development of tumor-induced T-cell anergy.[38–40]

NFATC2-rearranged sarcomas with *EWSR1* or *FUS* partners were provisionally categorized under the same subheading in the 2019 World Health Organization classification, noting, however, that the 2 groups appeared to be transcriptionally distinct on clustering analysis.[13,25] In addition, a recent study of 4 *NFATC2*-rearranged sarcomas analyzed by comparative genomic hybridization showed that those with *FUS::NFATC2* fusion had frequent deletions of tumor suppressor genes (including *CDKN2A/B*, *TUSC7*, and *DMD*) and more complex karyotypes than the *EWSR1::NFATC2* sarcomas; these findings could potentially be related to tumor biology, considering that all *FUS::NFATC2* sarcomas were clinically aggressive.[56] Collectively, these observations raise the question as to whether they should be categorized under the same umbrella or as distinct entities. Nevertheless, the number of cases reported, especially with the *FUS::NFATC2* fusion, is still too limited for definitive conclusions.[13,25,56]

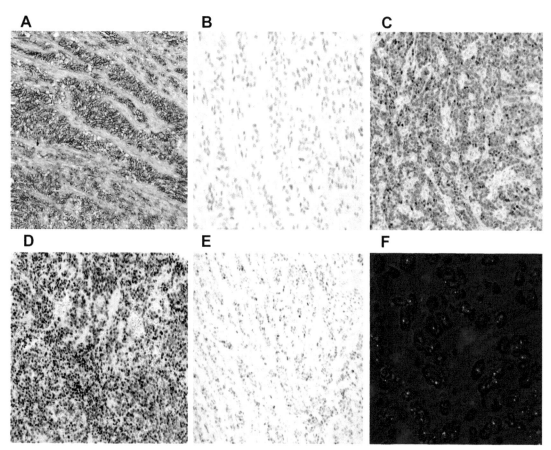

Fig. 6. *EWSR1::NFATC2* sarcoma with: (*A*) diffuse membranous CD99 expression; (*B*) moderate NKX2.2 nuclear immunoreactivity; (*C*) strong and diffuse PAX7 immunoreactivity; (*D*) strong and diffuse NKX3.1 expression; (*E*) strong and diffuse ETV4 nuclear immunoexpression, which can raise the differential of *CIC*-rearranged sarcoma; (*F*) *EWSR1* break-apart FISH analysis shows *EWSR1* rearrangement and amplification in an *EWSR1::NFATC2* sarcoma (×100). (Courtesy Dr. Akihiko Yoshida, Tokyo).

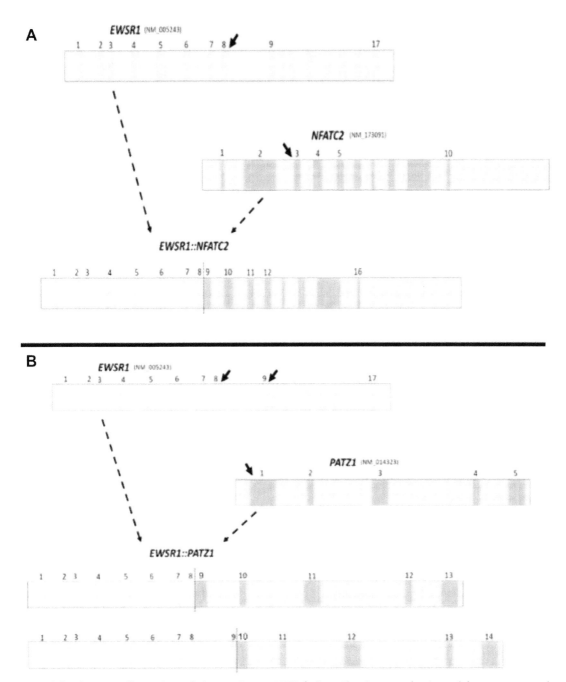

Fig. 7. (*A*) Schematic illustration of the *EWSR1::NFATC2* fusion. The 2 upper horizontal bars represent the genomic organization of the *EWSR1* and *NFATC2* genes. Blue and green solid boxes represent the exons (*numbered*), and the intronic regions are lightly shaded. The arrows indicate the fusion points. The 2 horizontal bars in the lower segment of the figure show the genomic structure of the *EWSR1::NFATC2* fusion gene. (*B*) Schematic illustration of the *EWSR1::PATZ1* fusion. The 2 upper horizontal bars represent the genomic organization of the *EWSR1* and *PATZ1* genes. Blue and green solid boxes represent the exons (*numbered*), and the intronic regions are lightly shaded. The arrows indicate the fusion points and show that exons 8 and 9 of *EWSR1* are fused to intraexonic sequences in the first exon of *PATZ1*. The 2 horizontal bars in the lower segment of the figure show the genomic structure of the *EWSR1::PATZ1* fusion genes.

Table 2
EWSR1::PATZ1

Study	Age/Gender	Location	Histopathology	IHC positive	IHC negative	Outcome	Follow-up months
Mastrangelo et al, 2000	16/M	Chest wall	Round cell sarcoma	SYN, NSE, desmin, keratin	CD99	AWD/Lung Mtx	24
Watson et al, 2018	0.9/M	Thigh	Malignant monomorphic spindle cell neoplasm	CD99, S100	Keratin, EMA	NR	NR
Watson et al, 2018	68/M	Subscapular	Malignant spindle cell neoplasm with hemangioma-like vasculature	CD99, S100	AE1/AE3, EMA	NR	NR
Watson et al, 2018	56/M	Mediastinum	Malignant epithelioid and spindle cell neoplasm	CD99, S100	Keratin, EMA	NR	NR
Watson et al, 2018	46/F	Paravertebral	Round cell sarcoma	NR	NR	NR	NR
Watson et al, 2018	32/M	Flank	Round cell sarcoma	NR	NR	NR	NR
Chougule et al, 2019	31/F	Retroperitoneal	Round and spindle cells, dense intratumoral fibrocollagenous stroma, necrosis	CD99, desmin, myogenin, MyoD1, S100, SOX10, CD34 and GFAP	AE1/AE3 and EMA	DOD/Lung and liver Mtx	5
Chougule et al, 2019	53/F	Right iliac fossa	Round and spindle cells, dense intratumoral fibrocollagenous stroma, no necrosis	CD99, Desmin, myogenin, MyoD1, S100, SOX10, CD34 and GFAP	AE1/AE3 and EMA	NED	3
Bridge et al, 2019	36/F	Chest wall	High grade small round blue cell tumor with fibrocollagenous bands	SYN, CD56, myogenin	S100, CK,EMA, GFAP	DOD	30
Bridge et al, 2019	53/F	Upper arm/axilla	Round and spindle cell morphology, fibrocollagen stroma, necrosis	SYN, S100, desmin, MyoD1, CD99, CD34, GFAP	SOX10, AE1/AE3, EMA	DOD	2
Bridge et al, 2019	81/F	Cervical neck	Round cells focally interrupted by cystic spaces and a myxohyaline background	S100, GFAP, desmin, CD99	SYN, SOX10, AE1/AE3, EMA, CD34	NED	19
Bridge et al, 2019	11/F	Chest wall	NR	NR	NR	NR	NR
Bridge et al, 2019	60/M	Chest wall	NR	NR	NR	NR	NR
Bridge et al, 2019	19/F	Head and neck	NR	NR	NR	NR	NR
Bridge et al, 2019	59/M	Lung	NR	NR	NR	NR	NR
Tsuda et al, 2020	ND/M	Extraskeletal/limb	Round/ovoid cell sarcoma	Desmin, MyoD1	NR	NR	NR
Tsuda et al, 2020	ND/M	Extraskeletal/limb	Round/ovoid cell sarcoma	NR	NR	NR	NR
Tsuda et al, 2020	ND/M	Extraskeletal/limb	Round/ovoid cell sarcoma	NR	NR	NR	NR
Michal et al, 2020	44/M	Abdominal wall	Low-grade spindle/round cell tumor, no necrosis, low mitotic index	S100, MyoD1, PAX7, AE1/AE3, MDM2, GFAP	Desmin, myogenin, SOX10, CD99, NKX2.2	NED	19
Michal et al, 2020	49/M	Rectus abdominal	Low-grade spindle/round cell tumor	S100, MyoD1, desmin, CD34, GFAP	AE1/AE3, SOX10, Synap, CK8/18, EMA	ND	ND
Michal et al, 2020	81/F	Posterior neck	Low-grade spindle/round cell tumor, hypercellular hyalinized stroma	S100, GFAP, desmin, MyoD1, PAX7	Myogenin, AE1/AE3, SOX10, CD99, NIKX2.2	AWUnknow	32
Michal et al, 2020	36/M	Abdominal wall	Low-grade spindle/round cell tumor, hypercellular hyalinized stroma	S100, GFAP, desmin, MyoD1, PAX7, AE1/AE3, SOX10	Myogenin, CD99, EMA, NKX2.2	NR	NR
Michal et al, 2020	10/F	Chest wall	Predominantly round cell sarcoma, microcystic appearance	S100, GFAP, desmin, MyoD1, AE1/AE3, CD99	Myogenin, CD34, SMA	NED	60
Michal et al, 2020	74/F	Lung, pleura	Predominantly round cell sarcoma, perimembranous collagen deposition	S100, CD99	Desmin, MyoD1, myogenin, AE1/AE3, SOX10	NR	NR
Michal et al, 2020	46/F	Abdominal wall	Predominantly round cell sarcoma, scarce stromal matrix	GFAP, desmin, MyoD1, SYN, caldesmon	S100, myogenin, AE1/AE3, CD99, SOX10	AWD/Lung Mtx	60
Michal et al, 2020	34/F	Trapezius muscle	High-grade spindle/round cell sarcoma, microcystic/reticular change, pleomorphism, fibrocollagenous tissue	S100, Desmin, MyoD1, PAX7, AE1/AE3, GFAP, MDM2	Myogenin, SOX10, CD99, NKX2.2, NKX3.1	AWD/Lung Mtx	18
Michal et al, 2020	66/M	Abdominal wall	High-grade spindle/round cell sarcoma, pleomorphism, fibrocollagenous tissue	Desmin, MyoD1, Myogenin, CD99, AE1/AE3	S100, GFAP, PAX7	AWD/Lung Mtx	ND
Park et al, 2020	52/F	Right neck	Small round cells with a trabecular pattern, hyalinized vessels and collagenous stroma	S100, GFAP, MyoD1, desmin	CD99, Pan-Keratin, CD34, SOX10	NED	ND
Wai Yau et al, 2021	5/M	Facial mass	High-grade spindle/round cell sarcoma, intercellular collagen, mitoses	S100, GFAP, SOX10, CD99, AE1/AE3, CK7	Desmin, MyoD1 and myogenin	AWD	36
Ngo et al, 2021	43/F	Retroperitoneal	High-grade round/ovoid/spindle cell sarcoma, high mitotic index	S100, SOX10, CD99, CD34	AE1/AE3, EMA, desmin, myogenin	ND	ND

Red, soft tissue location.
Abbreviations: AWUnknown, alive with unknown status; NSE, neuron specific enolase.

Various molecular approaches, such as NGS, fluorescence in situ hybridization (FISH), and reverse transcription polymerase chain reaction, can be used for the identification of the *EWSR1/FUS::NFATC2* fusion.[24–26,51–56] Detection of *EWSR1* rearrangement by FISH with concomitant amplification in the morphologic context of an undifferentiated round cell sarcoma is highly suggestive of *EWSR1::NFATC2* sarcoma.[24–26,51–56] It is important to remain aware, however, that the fusion is not entirely specific, as identical *EWSR1/FUS::NFATC2* fusions have been reported in simple bone cysts and osseous vascular tumors, albeit without *EWSR1* amplification.[60–64]

Differential Diagnosis

Undifferentiated round cell sarcomas (ES, *EWSR1::PATZ1* sarcoma, *BCOR*-altered, and *CIC*-rearranged sarcoma), extraskeletal myxoid chondrosarcoma (EMC), mesenchymal chondrosarcoma, myoepithelial tumor, metastatic carcinoma, and hematologic neoplasms all lie within the differential diagnosis of undifferentiated sarcomas harboring *EWSR1/FUS::NFATC2* fusions.[1,7,13,18–23,27–34,71–79]

ES shares the small round cell cytologic features and immunoreactivity for CD99, NKX2.2, and PAX7; however, it differs architecturally owing to its lack of a cohesive, cordlike or nested pattern.[1,6,7,13,15,16] Myxohyaline or extensive fibrotic/sclerotic stromal tissue is infrequent in ES.[18] Nevertheless, *EWSR1/FUS::NFATC2* sarcoma with limited stroma may create diagnostic difficulties by resembling ES, in which case NKX3.1 immunoreactivity would favor the former. A feature that may also be very helpful is the detection of *EWSR1* amplification by FISH, which is quite specific in the appropriate morphologic context for *EWSR1/FUS::NFATC2* sarcoma.[13,54,56]

EWSR1::PATZ1 sarcoma (discussed in greater detail in the next section) may display small, round, ovoid, or spindle-shaped cells and is often accompanied by a fibrous stroma with prominent

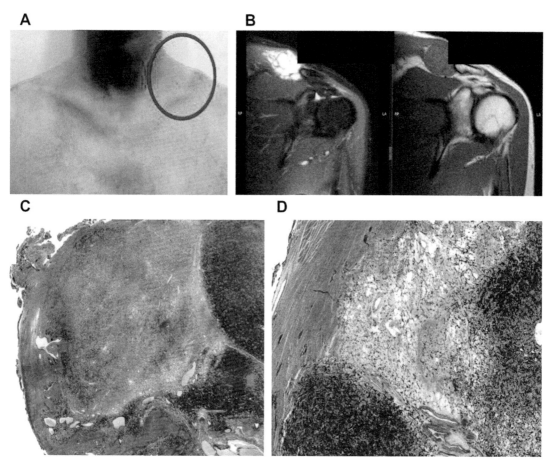

Fig. 8. (*A*) Chest wall/periclavicular mass. (*B*) MRI shows a large intramuscular mass in the left superior chest wall (trapezius muscle). Tumor location (*Circle*). (*C-D*) *EWSR1::PATZ1* sarcoma exhibiting well-circumscribed silhouette with variably thick fibrous capsule (H&E, original magnification ×200 and ×400).

perimembranous collagen accentuation.[80,81] Nearly all tumors exhibit coexpression of neural and myogenic markers, whereas NKX2.2 and NKX3.1 are negative. *EWSR1* amplification has not been reported in this type of sarcoma to date.[80–85]

BCOR-genetically altered sarcoma may share clinical features with *EWSR1/FUS::NFATC2* sarcoma, such as male predominance, osseous location, and younger age, as well as histologic and immunohistochemical similarities. BCOR immunohistochemistry is a sensitive but nonspecific marker that, along with cyclin B3, is diffusely expressed in most *BCOR::CCNB3* sarcomas.[27–34] The latter, however, is not expressed in other *BCOR* family tumors. Moreover, BCOR may also be expressed in some *EWSR1/FUS::NFATC2* sarcomas, rendering its assessment a less useful tool in this differential.[54–56] *EWSR1* FISH can be used to rule in/rule out the latter.

CIC-rearranged sarcoma usually shows higher-grade cytomorphology with prominent nucleoli, a high mitotic index, focal myxoid stromal tissue with variable CD99 expression, and ETV4 immunoreactivity.[19–26] Exceptionally, NKX3.1, NKX2.2, and AGGREGAN are expressed; however, the lack of *EWSR1* or *FUS* rearrangement is valuable to exclude an *EWSR1/FUS::NFATC2* sarcoma.[19–23] In difficult cases, FISH or targeted NGS, albeit with their own sensitivity limitations in this particular tumor, can be used to detect the diagnostic *CIC* fusions.

EMC may share similar histologic features, such as cordlike or nested growth patterns in chondromyxoid matrix[71–74], however, it is usually negative for CD99, NKX2.2, NKX3.1, and AGGREGAN.[54–58] In addition, in contrast to *EWSR1/FUS::NFATC2* sarcoma, neuroendocrine markers are frequently expressed in EMC.[71–74] *NR4A3* rearrangement is typical of EMC.[71–74]

The primitive round cell component of mesenchymal chondrosarcoma can express NKX3.1 and AGGRECAN, therefore, in a small biopsy with no cartilaginous component they have no

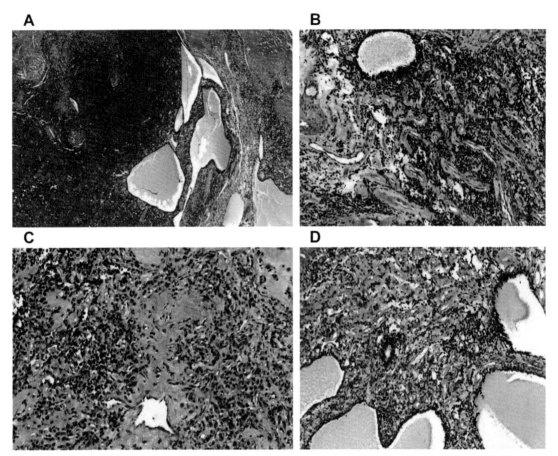

Fig. 9. (*A–D*) *EWSR1::PATZ1* sarcoma with multiple cystic structures and abundant fibrous stroma. (H&E, original magnification ×100 (*A*) and ×200 (*B-D*).

discriminatory value.[75–77] In contrast, PAX7 is frequently positive in *EWSR1/FUS::NFATC2* sarcoma, whereas it is usually negative in mesenchymal chondrosarcoma.[13,41,42,56] In difficult cases, the detection of the characteristic *HEY1::NCOA2* fusion can help confirm the latter.

EWSR1/FUS::NFATC2 sarcoma may express focal dotlike staining for keratin AE1/AE3 and CD138, raising the differential of metastatic carcinoma, myoepithelial tumor, or myeloma/plasmacytoma.[50–56] NKX3.1, which is a marker that is frequently used in the diagnosis of metastatic carcinoma of prostatic origin, is also positive in many *EWSR1/FUS::NFATC2* sarcomas. However, the keratin and EMA expression in the latter is not in a diffuse pattern as is seen in prostatic carcinoma.[50–56]

The differential diagnosis between a myoepithelial tumor and *EWSR1/FUS::NFATC2* sarcoma with cordlike or nested growth patterns, clear/epithelioid cells, fibrous or hyaline stromal tissue, and keratin/EMA expression may be challenging.[78,79] To complicate matters further, approximately 50% of myoepithelial tumors harbor *EWSR1* rearrangements (smaller subset harbor *FUS* rearrangement) and very rarely even *EWSR1* amplification and diffuse AGGRECAN expression.[13,56,78,79] NKX3.1 immunoreactivity can be helpful as, to the best of the authors' knowledge, it has not been reported in myoepithelial tumors.[54,55] The identification of the *EWSR1* or *FUS* fusion partner will definitively distinguish between the 2 entities.

Prognosis and Treatment

The clinical course of *EWSR1/FUS::NFATC2* sarcomas may include local recurrences and/or metastatic disease (reportedly to lung, bone, and skin).[13,54–56,59] Although in many patients disease control has been achieved with surgical resection, the histologic response to neoadjuvant therapy has been poor. The overall prognosis has been somewhat variable among studies.[13,54–56,59] In the Perret and colleagues series,[56] in 3 of 7 patients (42%) the clinical behavior was aggressive, including local recurrence, metastatic spread, and death.[56] Overall, ~42% of reported *EWSR1/*

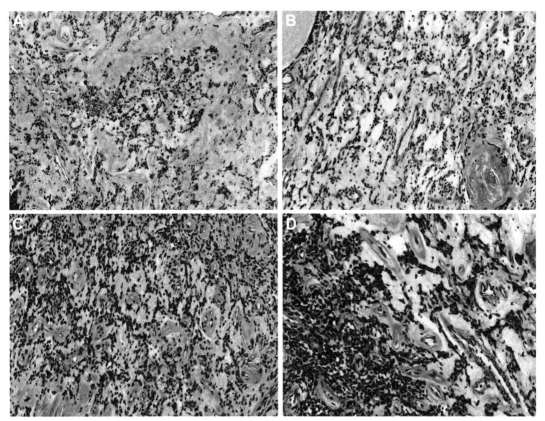

Fig. 10. (*A–B*) *EWSR1::PATZ1* sarcoma with low-grade features composed of bland round/ovoid cells with low mitotic index, lack of necrosis, and hyalinized/myxohyaline stromal tissue (H&E, original magnification ×200 and ×400). (*C-D*) *EWSR1::PATZ1* sarcoma with fibrous stroma and perimembranous collagen accentuation (H&E, original magnification ×200 and ×400).

FUS::NFATC2 sarcomas exhibited local recurrence or metastasis, similar to skeletal ES.[25,35–59] Data on the outcomes of *FUS::NFATC2* sarcoma specifically are very limited, although Perret and colleagues[56] suggested an even more aggressive behavior.

Interestingly, in a study published by Watson and colleagues,[25] the transcriptomes of *EWSR1::NFATC2* sarcomas were strongly enriched in genes associated with inflammatory and immune responses, while the transcriptomes of *FUS::NFATC2* sarcomas were enriched in proliferation and drug-resistance signatures. The aforementioned raises the possibility of exploring an immunotherapy approach for *EWSR1::N-FATC2* sarcomas and may explain the high mitotic index of *FUS::NFATC2* sarcomas, respectively.[25] In addition, Seligson and colleagues[59] conducted a multiscale-omic assessment of *EWSR1::NFATC2* fusion-positive sarcomas and identified the mTOR pathway as a potential therapeutic target. More specifically, they observed that *TOP1, TP53, NF1,* and *mTOR* variants helped define the *EWSR1::NFATC2* fusion-positive

samples.[59] Moreover, *STAG2,* a gene commonly altered in ES and associated with poor prognosis, was not altered in any subject with *EWSR1::N-FATC2* fusion.[59] These data reinforce previous findings regarding the unique nature of *EWSR1::NFATC2* sarcomas and associate these neoplasms with the activation of the mTOR pathway.[59] Prospective clinical evaluation will be required to validate whether mTOR inhibitor drugs could be a potential therapeutic target in *EWSR1::NFATC2* sarcomas.

In conclusion, *EWSR1/FUS::NFATC2* fusion-positive undifferentiated round cell sarcomas are uncommon, have distinct morphology, and are potentially biologically aggressive. It is important to recognize these entities, as they respond poorly to ES regimens, and new forms of therapy are needed.

SARCOMAS WITH *EWSR1::PATZ1* FUSION TRANSCRIPT

Background

EWSR1::PATZ1 sarcoma represents the second most frequent subtype of undifferentiated

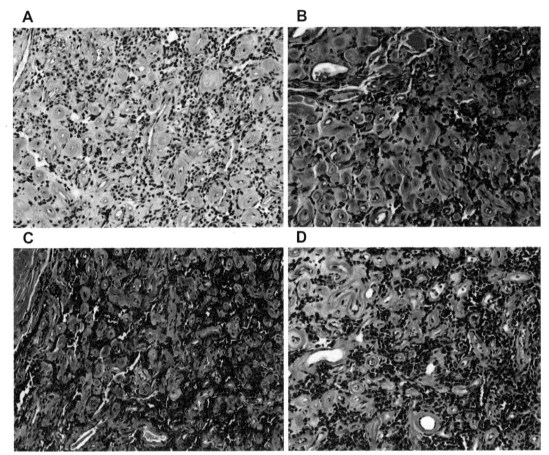

Fig. 11. (*A–D*) *EWSR1::PATZ1* sarcoma with low-grade features composed of round/ovoid cells with low mitotic index, hyalinized stromal tissue, and extensive perimembranous collagen accentuation (H&E, original magnification ×200 and ×400).

sarcoma with *EWSR1::non-ETS* fusions.[13,26,80–87] Considering the wide range of clinical and pathologic features observed in the Bridge and colleagues series[80] and prior reports,[13,26,81–87] it remains unclear whether *EWSR1::PATZ1* is a "disease-defining" fusion or a promiscuous genetic event that is present in several distinct mesenchymal neoplasms.[13,26,80–87] At the very least, this fusion can occur in sarcomas and primary central nervous system tumors, along with renal carcinomas.[65–70]

Clinical and Radiologic Findings

EWSR1::PATZ1 sarcomas affect patients with a wide age range (0.9–81 years) and similar sex distribution (**Table 2**). They typically arise in deep soft tissues with a predilection for the chest wall (**Fig. 8A–B**) and abdomen.[13,26,80–87] However, they have also been reported in other locations, such as the extremities (thigh and shoulder) and head/neck.[13,80,81] To the best of the authors' knowledge, no cases arising from the bone have been reported to date[13,26,80–87] (see **Table 2**). Patients with *EWSR1::PATZ1* sarcomas may present with a palpable soft tissue mass and/or pain related to tumor location and size or extent of disease. In a subset of cases, patients may present with distant or locoregional metastases at the time of diagnosis[13,80,81] (see **Table 2**).

Macroscopic Assessment and Histopathologic Features

Macroscopically, *EWSR1::PATZ1* sarcoma is typically a well-circumscribed, solid-cystic mass with or without necrosis and tan-yellow to gray-white cut surface. Its reported size ranges from 3.5 to over 10 cm in greatest dimension.[13,80,81]

The reported histologic features are wide-ranging, encompassing low-grade to high-grade neoplasms.[13,80,81] At low-power magnification,

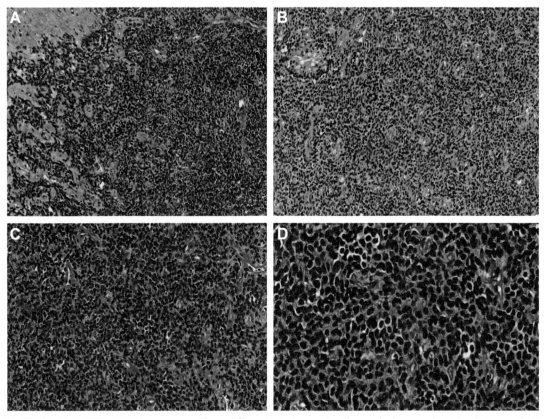

Fig. 12. (*A–D*) *EWSR1::PATZ1* sarcoma with undifferentiated round cell morphology and minimal stroma (H&E, original magnification ×200 (*A-C*) and ×400 (*D*).

the tumor may appear infiltrative or relatively well-circumscribed and partially encapsulated by a fibrous tissue of varying thickness[13,80,81] (see **Fig. 8**C-D). Irregular collagenous bands forming multiple lobules or cystic structures may be evident (**Fig. 9**A–D). Cytologically, the cells are small, round, ovoid, or spindle-shaped and often accompanied by a fibrous stroma and perimembranous collagen accentuation[80,81] (**Figs. 10–13**). Necrosis and mitotic activity may or may not be evident.[13,80,81] Michal and colleagues[81] reported 3 histologic subgroups in a large series of *EWSR1::PATZ1* sarcomas. The first group had a low-grade appearance with round, ovoid, spindle, or epithelioid cells, a low mitotic index, absent necrosis, and hyalinized or myxohyaline stroma.[81] The second group was composed of round cells with minimal stromal matrix, and the third group exhibited high-grade spindle/round cell sarcoma morphology.[81]

Immunoprofile

Almost all tumors show coexpression of neural and myogenic markers.[13,26,80–87] Most tumors are S100-protein and GFAP immunoreactive (**Fig. 14**A–B), although some may show positivity for SOX10 and MITF as well.[13,80,81] Desmin, MyoD1 (see **Fig. 14**C–D), and PAX7 are the most commonly expressed myogenic markers, whereas myogenin is positive in some tumors.[13,80,81] Keratin (AE1/AE3) expression, predominantly with a dotlike perinuclear pattern, has been reported; CD34, smooth muscle actin, H-caldesmon, MDM2, and synaptophysin can also be positive.[13,80,81] Some tumors may show loss of nuclear H3K27me3 expression,[13,80,81] whereas CD99 immunoreactivity is occasionally observed (see **Fig 14**C), but the staining pattern is usually not as strong or membranous as observed in ES. EMA, BCOR, NKX2.2, NKX3.1, STAT6, and SSX::SS18 are negative.[13,80,81]

Genetic Features

As *EWSR1* and *PATZ1* genes are localized in close proximity to each other on chromosome 22 and are normally transcribed in opposite directions, the *EWSR1::PATZ1* fusion event is most likely the result of a cryptic intrachromosomal

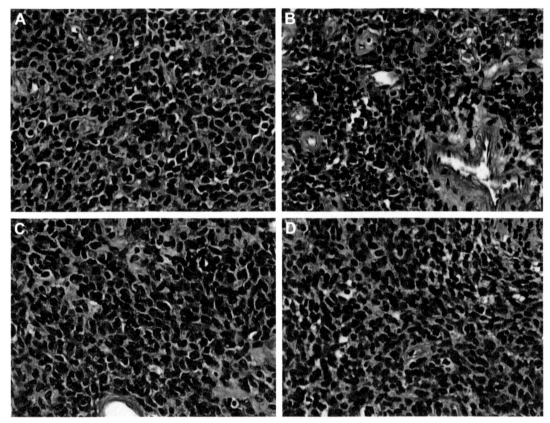

Fig. 13. (A–D) *EWSR1::PATZ1* sarcoma with undifferentiated round cell morphology, exhibiting hyperchromatic nuclei and some bizarre forms (H&E, original magnification ×400).

paracentric inversion[13,80,81] (**Fig. 7B**). Hence, the sensitivity of *EWSR1* break-apart FISH is low (see **Fig 14F**), and additional molecular studies (such as NGS) are required to identify this specific gene fusion.[13,80,81] In general, this highlights the potential limitation of using break-apart FISH probes in tumors with cryptic insertions or translocations as has also been observed in sarcomas with *BCOR::CCNB3* fusion, solitary fibrous tumor with *NAB2::STAT6* fusion, a subset of *CIC*-fusion sarcomas, or, rarely, in ES with *EWSR1:ERG* fusion.[17,32] Of note, however, fusion FISH probe sets may be used to detect some of these fusions.[17,32]

In some studies, the loss of *CDKN2A* in ES has been linked to highly aggressive behavior and poor response to chemotherapy.[1–7] Interestingly, Bridge and colleagues[80] reported in their series loss or partial deletion of *CDKN2A/CDKN2B* in 71% of tumors with *EWSR1::PATZ1* fusion. More specifically, both cases with metastatic disease upon presentation and poor therapeutic responses harbored *CDKN2A/CDKN2B* alterations, in contrast to another case that lacked this secondary genetic change and was clinically indolent.[80] Moreover, one of the cases with homozygous deletion of the 9p21.3 locus (*CDKN2A*) also showed concurrent *MDM2* amplification, which may also be associated with poor prognosis.[80]

Gene expression profiling analysis of small round cell sarcomas has shown that those with *EWSR1::PATZ1* fusion form a distinct separate tight cluster.[13,24–26,59,80,81] Additional transcriptional studies have also demonstrated that *EWSR1::PATZ1* sarcomas cluster tightly together and separate from other *EWSR1*-fused tumors, indicating a transcriptionally different entity.[24–26]

Differential Diagnosis

Depending on the predominant tumor morphology, *EWSR1::PATZ1* sarcomas with spindle, round, or ovoid/epithelioid cells, morphologically may resemble various mesenchymal neoplasms (malignant peripheral nerve sheath tumor [MPNST], synovial sarcoma/SS, ossifying fibromyxoid tumor, solitary fibrous tumor/SFT), other undifferentiated round cell sarcomas, *GLI1*-altered neoplasm, or myoepithelial tumor/carcinoma.[13,80,81,88–101]

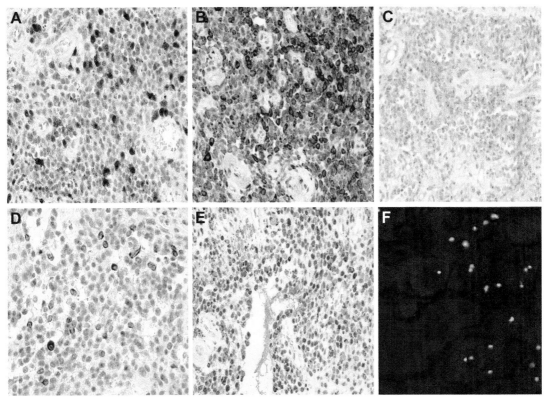

Fig. 14. *EWSR1::PATZ1* sarcoma. (*A*) Patchy and nuclear S100 immunoreactivity. (*B*) Strong and diffuse GFAP positivity. (*C*) Dot-like CD99 expression. (*D*) Focal and cytoplasmic desmin expression. (*E*) Strong and diffuse MyoD1 immunoreactivity. (*F*) *EWSR1* break-apart FISH demonstrating lack of a rearrangement with orange and green flanking probes remaining juxtaposed (less than a signal size apart).

Immunohistochemically, although S100 protein and keratin (AE1/AE3) expression may cause confusion with myoepithelial carcinoma, immunoreactivity for neural and myogenic/rhabdomyoblastic markers would support the diagnosis of *EWSR1::PATZ1* sarcoma.[13,78–81] The presence of fascicular growth pattern with some keratin positivity may suggest the diagnosis of synovial sarcoma, which can be easily distinguished by detecting its characteristic *SS18::SSX* fusion.[92,93] MPNST with rhabdomyoblastic differentiation can potentially be a challenging differential, and the clinical history of neurofibromatosis 1 would be helpful.[88–90] Conversely, some cases of *EWSR1::PATZ1* sarcoma with predominant spindle cells may resemble an MPNST with rhabdomyoblastic differentiation, and intriguingly in one of 2 molecularly confirmed *EWSR1::PATZ1* sarcomas, there was near-complete loss of H3K27me2 nuclear expression.[81] Interestingly, one case of MPNST (reportedly) with *EWSR1::-VEZF1* fusion showed a similar morphology but had a different immunoprofile with positive expression of desmin, myogenin, SOX10, and EMA, and

lack of S100/GFAP and keratin immunoreactivity.[91]

Although typical ES is composed of monotonous round cells, the atypical variant may show a partial spindle/ovoid cell morphology resembling an *EWSR1::PATZ1* sarcoma. The latter may occasionally show membranous CD99 expression, but diffuse and strong membranous positivity as seen in ES is not observed.[13,80,81] Moreover, NKX2.2, which is usually expressed in ES, is negative in *EWSR1::PATZ1* sarcomas.[13,80,81] Immunoreactivity for myogenic markers is an extremely rare event in ES.[1–6] *BCOR*-genetically altered and *CIC*-rearranged sarcomas may also show spindle and round cell morphology, but generally they do not express desmin or S100 protein.[19–23,27–34] In desmoplastic small round cell tumor, S100/GFAP expression and MyoD1 immunoreactivity are usually absent, whereas nuclear WT1 expression (C-terminus) has not been reported in *EWSR1::PATZ1* sarcomas.[13,80,81]

Because of the expression of myogenic/rhabdomyoblastic markers, naturally the diagnosis of RMS enters the differential. Although the latter

Table 3
Clinical and morphologic features

	Patient Characteristics	Location	Round/Ovoid Cells	Spindle or Pleomorphic Cells	Clear/Epithelioid/Rhabdoid Cells	Sclerotic/Fibrotic Stroma	Cordlike Pattern	Myxohyaline Stroma	Cytoplasm	Perimembranous Collagen Deposits	Prognosis/Survival/Outcome/Treatment
Ewing sarcoma (ES)	1st to 2nd decade	85% diaphysis-metaphysis long bones > pelvis, ribs chest wall. 15% extraskeletal/soft tissue (adults)	Yes	Rare	Occasional	Rare	Rare	Rare	Scant	Rare	Local recurrence and systemic metastases (lung, bone). Surgery and/or radiation (local control). Chemotherapy (ES regimen)
EWSR1/FUS::NFATC2 sarcoma	Strong male predilection. 4th decade (older than ES)	Long bones > soft tissue (4:1) *FUS::NFATC2*: long bones	Yes	Occasional	Yes	Variable	Frequent	Frequent	Variable	Focal	Local recurrence and systemic metastases (lung, cutaneous, and bone). Surgery and/or radiation (local control). Chemotherapy (ES regimen with poor response)
EWSR1::PATZ1 sarcoma	4th decade	Soft tissue/chest wall, head and neck	Yes	Yes	Rare	Variable	Rare	Variable	Variable	Yes and prominent	Metastases. Surgery and/or radiation (local control). Chemotherapy (ES regimen with limited response)

Table 4
Immunohistochemical and molecular findings

	CD99	NKX2.2	PAX7	NKX3.1	Keratin/ EMA	Myogenic Marker	S100 /SOX10/ GFAP	SMA	FISH EWSR1	Gene Fusions	Additional Molecular Alterations	Potential Differential Diagnoses
Ewing sarcoma (ES)	SD	SDN	neg		20%–30%	Very rare	Rare	V	Translocation/no amplification	*EWSR1:ETS* (*FLI1, ERG, FEV, ETV1, E1AF*)	STAG2 mutation, CDKN2A/TP53 mutation	Undifferentiated round cell sarcomas (*EWSR1/ FUS::NFATC2* sarcoma, *CIC*-rearranged sarcoma, *EWSR1::PATZ1* sarcoma, *BCOR*-associated sarcoma), rhabdomyosarcoma, neuroblastoma, myeloma/lymphoma, melanoma, metastatic carcinomas
EWSR1/FUS:: NFATC2 sarcoma	V	SDN	SDN		Poor/dot-like	Very rare	Rare	V	Translocation and amplification	*EWSR1::NFATC2 FUS::NFATC2*	CDKN2A/B, TUSC7, and/or DMD deletion in *FUS* rearranged tumor	Ewing sarcoma and other undifferentiated round cell sarcomas (eg, *BCOR*-associated sarcomas), mesenchymal chondrosarcoma, myoepithelial tumors, metastatic carcinoma (mainly of prostatic origin), extraskeletal myxoid chondrosarcoma, hematologic neoplasms (plasmacytoma/myeloma/ lymphoma)
EWSR1:: PATZ1 sarcoma	V	Neg	Neg		Poor/dot-like	Positive	++	V	Low sensitivity	*EWSR1::PATZ1*	CDKN2A/CDKN2B deletion. MDM2 amplification	Ewing sarcoma and other undifferentiated round cell sarcomas (*BCOR*-associated sarcoma, *CIC*-rearranged sarcoma, *EWSR1/ FUS::NFATC2* sarcoma), MPNST, synovial sarcoma, ossifying fibromyxoid tumor, solitary fibrous tumor, or myoepithelial neoplasms.

Abbreviations: Neg, negative; SD, strong/diffuse and membranous; SDN, nuclear; strong and diffuse; V, variable.

may have spindle cell morphology, at the cytogenetic level most cases of RMS do not harbor *EWSR1* gene rearrangements.[102–105] However, a recently described rare subset with bone predominance, round/epithelioid/spindle cell morphology, and frequent ALK expression has been reported to harbor the *EWSR1/FUS::TFCP2* gene fusion.[103]

Prognosis and Treatment

Previous publications have emphasized the very aggressive clinical behavior of most *EWSR1::-PATZ1* sarcomas, with patients either dying or developing distant metastases within 2 to 60 months of follow-up[13,26,80–87] (see **Table 2**). In addition, the response to conventional systemic chemotherapies has been poor and does not seem to provide any clinical benefit, although the limited number of patients precludes definite conclusions.

Preliminary data suggest that there may be an association between morphologic features and clinical behavior. In particular, well-circumscribed or partially encapsulated tumors with scarce mitotic activity and low-grade morphology may behave less aggressively.[13,80,81] At the molecular level, the presence of copy number loss or deletion of *CDKN2A/CDKN2B* genes and *MDM2* gene amplification seems to be related to poor prognosis. Furthermore, *TP53* mutation has also been reported in tumors with aggressive morphology and may have potential prognostic relevance.[13,80,81]

Surgical resection remains the mainstay of treatment, whereas patients with metastatic disease experience poor response or resistance to conventional systemic chemotherapies in the neoadjuvant or adjuvant setting.[13] Data on radiotherapy are limited.

The presence of *MDM2* amplification and *CDKN2A/B* deletion may suggest the potential utility of targeted therapy, such as CDK4/6 inhibitors, although these alterations are not present in all cases.[80] In a previous study of 6 cases of *EWSR1::PATZ1* sarcomas, these tumors clustered separately from classic ES by gene expression analysis; notable differences in gene expression include high levels of *GPR12*, a G protein–coupled receptor.[25] Interestingly, GPR12 has been shown to bind to sphingosine-1-phosphate as its predicted ligand, and its activity could potentially be modulated by phytocannabinoid cannabidiol.[25] Further studies of the sphingosine-1-phosphate/G protein–coupled receptor axis may open up new treatment strategies for this group of sarcomas.

Tables **3** and **4** summarize the morphologic, immunohistochemical, and molecular features of *EWSR1/FUS::NFATC2* and *EWSR1::PATZ1* sarcomas.

CLINICS CARE POINTS

- *EWSR1/FUS::NFATC2* and *EWSR1::PATZ1* sarcomas have been reported not only in malignant soft tissue tumors but also in unrelated benign entities of different lineages, reinforcing the imperfect diagnostic specificity of these gene fusions and highlighting the importance of correlating histologic, immunohistochemical, and genetic findings with clinical data.

- DNA methylation-based classification and gene expression analysis have further demonstrated that *EWSR1/FUS::NFATC2* and *EWSR1::PATZ1* sarcomas are genetically and epigenetically distinct from classic Ewing sarcoma.

- The clinical course of *EWSR1::NFATC2* sarcomas may include local recurrences and/or metastatic spread. Outcome data for *FUS::N-FATC2* sarcomas are still limited, however, they suggest an even more aggressive behavior.

- *EWSR1/FUS::NFATC2* sarcomas show poor to no response to conventional neoadjuvant chemotherapy.

- The transcriptomes of *EWSR1::NFATC2* sarcomas are enriched in genes associated with inflammatory and immune responses, suggesting the possibility of exploring an immunotherapy approach. Moreover, the mTOR pathway has been identified as a potential therapeutic target for *EWSR1::NFATC2* sarcomas.

- *EWSR1::PATZ1* sarcomas frequently exhibit very aggressive clinical behavior, with reports indicating that patients either die or develop distant metastases within a short time period.

- Surgical resection remains the mainstay of treatment for *EWSR1::PATZ1* sarcomas. Patients experience poor responses or resistance to conventional systemic chemotherapies in the neoadjuvant or adjuvant therapy settings.

DISCLOSURE

The authors have nothing to disclose.

REFERENCES

1. Antonescu C. Round cell sarcomas beyond Ewing: emerging entities. Histopathology 2014;64:26–37.

2. Ohno T, Ouchida M, Lee L, et al. The EWS gene, involved in Ewing family of tumors, malignant melanoma of soft parts and desmoplastic small round cell tumors, codes for an RNA binding protein with novel regulatory domains. Oncogene 1994;9:3087–97.

3. Tirode F, Surdez D, Ma X, et al. Genomic landscape of Ewing sarcoma defines an aggressive subtype with co-association of STAG2 and TP53 mutations. Cancer Discov 2014;4:1342–53.

4. Crompton BD, Stewart C, Taylor-Weiner A, et al. The genomic landscape of pediatric Ewing sarcoma. Cancer Discov 2014;4:1326–41.

5. Mantilla JG, Ricciotti RW, Chen E, et al. Detecting disease-defining gene fusions in unclassified round cell sarcomas using anchored multiplex PCR/targeted RNA next-generation sequencing-Molecular and clinicopathological characterization of 16 cases. Genes Chromosomes Cancer 2019;58:713–22.

6. Tsuda Y, Zhang L, Meyers P, et al. The clinical heterogeneity of round cell sarcomas with EWSR1/FUS gene fusions: Impact of gene fusion type on clinical features and outcome. Genes Chromosomes Cancer 2020;59:525–34.

7. Miettinen M, Felisiak-Golabek A, Luiña Contreras A, et al. New fusion sarcomas: histopathology and clinical significance of selected entities. Hum Pathol 2019;86:57–65.

8. Lam SW, Cleton-Jansen AM, Cleven AHG, et al. Molecular Analysis of gene fusions in bone and soft tissue tumors by anchored multiplex PCR-based targeted next-generation sequencing. J Mol Diagn 2018;20:653–63.

9. Szurian K, Kashofer K, Liegl-Atzwanger B. Role of next-generation sequencing as a diagnostic tool for the evaluation of bone and soft-tissue tumors. Pathobiology 2017;84:323–38.

10. Scolnick JA, Dimon M, Wang IC, et al. An efficient method for identifying gene fusions by targeted RNA sequencing from fresh frozen and FFPE samples. PLoS One 2015;10:e0128916.

11. Mertens F, Tayebwa J. Evolving techniques for gene fusion detection in soft tissue tumours. Histopathology 2014;64:151–62.

12. Beck AH, West RB, van de Rijn M. Gene expression profiling for the investigation of soft tissue sarcoma pathogenesis and the identification of diagnostic, prognostic, and predictive biomarkers. Virchows Arch 2010;456:141–51.

13. Le Loarer F, Szuhai K, Tirode F. Round cell sarcoma with EWSR1-non ETS fusion. In: WHO, classification of tumours of soft tissue and bone. 5th Edition. Lyon, France: IARC; 2019. p. 326–9.

14. Neuville A, Ranchère-Vince D, Dei Tos AP, et al. Impact of molecular analysis on the final sarcoma diagnosis: a study on 763 cases collected during a European epidemiological study. Am J Surg Pathol 2013;37:1259–68.

15. Sankar S, Lessnick SL. Promiscuous partnerships in Ewing's sarcoma. Cancer Genet 2011;204:351–65.

16. Brohl AS, Solomon DA, Chang W, et al. The genomic landscape of the Ewing Sarcoma family of tumors reveals recurrent STAG2 mutation. PLoS Genet 2014;10:e1004475.

17. Chen S, Deniz K, Sung YS, et al. Ewing sarcoma with ERG gene rearrangements: A molecular study focusing on the prevalence of FUS-ERG and common pitfalls in detecting EWSR1-ERG fusions by FISH. Genes Chromosomes Cancer 2016;55:340–9.

18. Thway K, Fisher C. Mesenchymal Tumors with EWSR1 Gene Rearrangements. Surg Pathol Clin 2019;12:165–90.

19. Antonescu CR, Owosho AA, Zhang L, et al. Sarcomas with CIC-rearrangements are a distinct pathologic entity with aggressive outcome: a clinicopathologic and molecular study of 115 cases. Am J Surg Pathol 2017;41:941–9.

20. Italiano A, Sung YS, Zhang L, et al. High prevalence of CIC fusion with double-homeobox (DUX4) transcription factors in EWSR1-negative undifferentiated small blue round cell sarcomas. Genes Chromosomes Cancer 2012;51:207–18.

21. Yoshida A, Goto K, Kodaira M, et al. CIC-rearranged sarcomas: a study of 20 cases and comparisons with Ewing sarcomas. Am J Surg Pathol 2016;40:313–23.

22. Gambarotti M, Benini S, Gamberi G, et al. CIC-DUX4 fusion-positive round-cell sarcomas of soft tissue and bone: a single-institution morphological and molecular analysis of seven cases. Histopathology 2016;69:624–34.

23. Yoshida A, Arai Y, Kobayashi E, et al. CIC break-apart fluorescence in-situ hybridization misses a subset of CIC-DUX4 sarcomas: a clinicopathological and molecular study. Histopathology 2017;71:461–9.

24. Specht K, Sung YS, Zhang L, et al. Distinct transcriptional signature and immunoprofile of CIC::-DUX4 fusion-positive round cell tumors compared to EWSR1-rearranged Ewing sarcomas: further evidence toward distinct pathologic entities. Genes Chromosomes Cancer 2014;53:622–33.

25. Watson S, Perrin V, Guillemot D, et al. Transcriptomic definition of molecular subgroups of small round cell sarcomas. J Pathol 2018;245(1):29–40.

26. Koelsche C, Kriegsmann M, Kommoss FKF, et al. DNA methylation profiling distinguishes Ewing-like sarcoma with EWSR1-NFATc2 fusion from Ewing sarcoma. J Cancer Res Clin Oncol 2019;145: 1273–81.

27. Pierron G, Tirode F, Lucchesi C, et al. A new sub-type of bone sarcoma defined by BCOR-CCNB3 gene fusion. Nat Gen 2012;44:461–6.

28. Cohen-Gogo S, Cellier C, Coindre JM, et al. Ewing-like sarcomas with BCOR-CCNB3 fusion transcript: a clinical, radiological and pathological retrospective study from the Société Française des cancers de L'Enfant. Pediatr Blood Cancer 2014;61:2191–8.

29. Puls F, Niblett A, Marland G, et al. BCOR-CCNB3 (Ewing-like) sarcoma: a clinicopathologic analysis of 10 cases, in comparison with conventional Ewing sarcoma. Am J Surg Pathol 2014;38:1307–18.

30. Li WS, Liao IC, Wen MC, et al. BCOR-CCNB3-positive soft tissue sarcoma with round-cell and spindle-cell histology: a series of four cases highlighting the pitfall of mimicking poorly differentiated synovial sarcoma. Histopathology 2016;69: 792–801.

31. Matsuyama A, Shiba E, Umekita Y, et al. Clinicopathologic diversity of undifferentiated sarcoma with BCOR-CCNB3 fusion: analysis of 11 cases with a reappraisal of the utility of immunohistochemistry for BCOR and CCNB3. Am J Surg Pathol 2017;41:1713–21.

32. Kao YC, Owosho AA, Sung YS, et al. BCOR-CCNB3 fusion positive sarcomas: a clinicopathologic and molecular analysis of 36 cases with comparison to morphologic spectrum and clinical behavior of other round cell sarcomas. Am J Surg Pathol 2018;42:604–15.

33. Yamada Y, Kuda M, Kohashi K, et al. Histological and immunohistochemical characteristics of undifferentiated small round cell sarcomas associated with CIC-DUX4 and BCOR-CCNB3 fusion genes. Virchows Arch 2017;470:373–80.

34. Kao YC, Sung YS, Zhang L, et al. BCOR overexpression is a highly sensitive marker in round cell sarcomas with BCOR genetic abnormalities. Am J Surg Pathol 2016;40:1670–8.

35. Ishida T, Kikuchi F, Oka T, et al. Case report 727. Juxtacortical adamantinoma of humerus (simulating Ewing tumor). Skeletal Radiol 1992;21:205–9.

36. Szuhai K, Ijszenga M, de Jong D, et al. The NFATc2 gene is involved in a novel cloned translocation in a Ewing sarcoma variant that couples its function in immunology to oncology. Clin Cancer Res 2009; 15:2259–68.

37. Wang WL, Patel NR, Caragea M, et al. Expression of ERG, an Ets family transcription factor, identifies ERG-rearranged Ewing sarcoma. Mod Pathol 2012; 25:1378–83.

38. Jauliac S, Lopez-Rodriguez C, Shaw LM, et al. The role of NFAT transcription factors in integrin-mediated carcinoma invasion. Nat Cell Biol 2002; 4:540–4.

39. Zhang X, Zhang Z, Cheng J, et al. Transcription factor NFAT1 activates the mdm2 oncogene independent of p53. J Biol Chem 2012;287:30468–76.

40. Lang T, Ding X, Kong L, et al. NFATC2 is a novel therapeutic target for colorectal cancer stem cells. OncoTargets Ther 2018;11:6911–24.

41. Charville GW, Wang WL, Ingram DR, et al. EWSR1 fusion proteins mediate PAX7 expression in Ewing sarcoma. Mod Pathol 2017;30:1312–20.

42. Charville GW, Wang WL, Ingram DR, et al. PAX7 expression in sarcomas bearing the EWSR1-NFATC2 translocation. Mod Pathol 2019;32:154–6.

43. Brcic I, Scheipl S, Bergovec M, et al. Implementation of Copy Number Variations-Based Diagnostics in Morphologically Challenging EWSR1/FUS::NFATC2 Neoplasms of the Bone and Soft Tissue. Int J Mol Sci 2022;23:16196.

44. Romeo S, Bovée JV, Kroon HM, et al. Malignant fibrous histiocytoma and fibrosarcoma of bone: a re-assessment in the light of currently employed morphological, immunohistochemical and molecular approaches. Virchows Arch 2012;461:561–70.

45. Sadri N, Barroeta J, Pack SD, et al. Malignant round cell tumor of bone with EWSR1-NFATC2 gene fusion. Virchows Arch 2014;465(2):233–9.

46. Kinkor Z, Vaneček T, Svajdler M Jr, et al. Where does Ewing sarcoma end and begin - two cases of unusual bone tumors with t(20;22)(EWSR1-NFATc2) alteration. Cesk Patol 2014;50:87–91.

47. Cohen JN, Sabnis AJ, Krings G, et al. EWSR1-NFATC2 gene fusion in a soft tissue tumor with epithelioid round cell morphology and abundant stroma: a case report and review of the literature. Hum Pathol 2018;81:281–90.

48. Baldauf MC, Gerke JS, Orth MF, et al. Are EWSR1-NFATc2-positive sarcomas really Ewing sarcomas? Mod Pathol 2018;31:997–9.

49. Toki S, Wakai S, Sekimizu M, et al. PAX7 immunohistochemical evaluation of Ewing sarcoma and other small round cell tumours. Histopathology 2018;73:645–52.

50. Yau DTW, Chan JKC, Bao S, et al. Bone Sarcoma With EWSR1-NFATC2 Fusion: Sarcoma With Varied Morphology and Amplification of Fusion Gene Distinct From Ewing Sarcoma. Int J Surg Pathol 2019;27:561–7.

51. Bode-Lesniewska B, Fritz C, Exner GU, et al. EWSR1-NFATC2 and FUS-NFATC2 Gene Fusion-Associated Mesenchymal Tumors: Clinicopathologic Correlation and Literature Review. Sarcoma 2019;26:9386390.

52. Wang GY, Thomas DG, Davis JL, et al. EWSR1-NFATC2 Translocation-associated Sarcoma Clinicopathologic Findings in a Rare Aggressive Primary Bone or Soft Tissue Tumor. Am J Surg Pathol 2019;43:1112–22.

53. Diaz-Perez JA, Nielsen GP, Antonescu C, et al. EWSR1/FUS-NFATc2 rearranged round cell sarcoma: clinicopathological series of 4 cases and literature review. Hum Pathol 2019;90:45–53.

54. Yoshida KI, Machado I, Motoi T, et al. NKX3-1 Is a Useful Immunohistochemical Marker of EWSR1-NFATC2 Sarcoma and Mesenchymal Chondrosarcoma. Am J Surg Pathol 2020;44:719–28.

55. Yoshida A, Hashimoto T, Ryo E, et al. Confirmation of NKX3-1 expression in EWSR1-NFATC2 sarcoma and mesenchymal chondrosarcoma using monoclonal antibody immunohistochemistry, RT-PCR, and RNA in situ hybridization. Am J Surg Pathol 2021;45:578–82.

56. Perret R, Escuriol J, Velasco V, et al. NFATc2-rearranged sarcomas: clinicopathologic, molecular, and cytogenetic study of 7 cases with evidence of AGGRECAN as a novel diagnostic marker. Mod Pathol 2020;33:1930–44.

57. Makise N, Yoshida KI, Iijima T, et al. Skeletal EWSR1-NFATC2 sarcoma previously diagnosed as Ewing-like adamantinoma: A case report and literature review emphasizing its unique radiological features. Pathol Int 2021;71:614–20.

58. Tsuchie H, Umakoshi M, Hasegawa T, et al. Soft tissue round cell sarcoma of the abdominal wall, with EWSR1-non-ETS fusion (EWSR1-NFATC2 sarcoma): A case report and literature review emphasizing its clinical features. J Orthop Sci 2022;13:S0949–2658.

59. Seligson ND, Maradiaga RD, Stets CM, et al. Multiscale-omic assessment of EWSR1-NFATc2 fusion positive sarcomas identifies the mTOR pathway as a potential therapeutic target. NPJ Precis Oncol 2021;5:43.

60. Shaheen M, Wurtz D, Brocken E, et al. EWSR1::NFATC2-rearranged sarcoma in bone-case report and review of the literature. Human Pathology Reports 2022;30:30068.

61. Pizem J, Sekoranja D, Zupan A, et al. FUS-NFATC2 or EWSR1-NFATC2 fusions are present in a large proportion of simple bone cysts. Am J Surg Pathol 2020;44:1623–34.

62. Hung YP, Fisch AS, Diaz-Perez JA, et al. Identification of EWSR1-NFATC2 fusion in simple bone cysts. Histopathology 2020;78:849–56.

63. Arbajian E, Magnusson L, Brosjo O, et al. A benign vascular tumor with a new fusion gene: EWSR1-NFATC1 in hemangioma of the bone. Am J Surg Pathol 2013;37:613–6 - PubMed.

64. Ong SLM, Lam SW, van den Akker BEWM, et al. Expanding the Spectrum of EWSR1-NFATC2-rearranged Benign Tumors: A Common Genomic Abnormality in Vascular Malformation/Hemangioma and Simple Bone Cyst. Am J Surg Pathol 2021;45:1669–81.

65. Siegfried A, Rousseau A, Maurage CA, et al. EWSR1-PATZ1 gene fusion may define a new glioneuronal tumor entity. Brain Pathol 2019;29:53–62.

66. Alhalabi KT, Stichel D, Sievers P, et al. PATZ1 fusions define a novel molecularly distinct neuroepithelial tumor entity with a broad histological spectrum. Acta Neuropathol 2021;142:841–57.

67. Rossi S, Barresi S, Giovannoni I, et al. Expanding the spectrum of EWSR1-PATZ1 rearranged CNS tumors: An infantile case with leptomeningeal dissemination. Brain Pathol 2021;31:e12934.

68. Lopez-Nunez O, Cafferata B, Santi M, et al. The spectrum of rare central nervous system (CNS) tumors with EWSR1-non-ETS fusions: experience from three pediatric institutions with review of the literature. Brain Pathol 2021;31:70–83.

69. Al-Obaidy KI, Bridge JA, Cheng L, et al. EWSR1-PATZ1 fusion renal cell carcinoma: a recurrent gene fusion characterizing thyroid-like follicular renal cell carcinoma. Mod Pathol 2021;34:1921–34.

70. Perret R, Lefort F, Bernhard JC, et al. Thyroid-like follicular renal cell carcinoma with sarcomatoid differentiation and an aggressive clinical course: a case report confirming the presence of the EWSR1::PATZ1 fusion gene. Histopathology 2022;80:745–8.

71. Rubin BP, Fletcher JA. Skeletal and extraskeletal myxoid chondrosarcoma: related or distinct tumors? Adv Anat Pathol 1999;6:204–12.

72. Panagopoulos I, Mertens F, Isaksson M, et al. Molecular genetic characterization of the EWS/CHN and RBP56/CHN fusion genes in extraskeletal myxoid chondrosarcoma. Genes Chromosomes Cancer 2002;35:340–52.

73. Yoshida A, Makise N, Wakai S, et al. INSM1 expression and its diagnostic significance in extraskeletal myxoid chondrosarcoma. Mod Pathol 2018;31:744–52.

74. Sugino H, Iwata S, Satomi K, et al. Keratin-positive fibrotic extraskeletal myxoid chondrosarcoma: a close mimic of myoepithelial tumour. Histopathology 2023;82:937–45.

75. Granter SR, Renshaw AA, Fletcher CD, et al. CD99 reactivity in mesenchymal chondrosarcoma. Hum Pathol 1996;27:1273–6.

76. Xu B, Rooper LM, Dermawan JK, et al. Mesenchymal chondrosarcoma of the head and neck with HEY1::NCOA2 fusion: A clinicopathologic and molecular study of 13 cases with emphasis on diagnostic pitfalls. Genes Chromosomes Cancer 2022;61:670–7.

77. Syed M, Mushtaq S, Loya A, et al. NKX3.1 a useful marker for mesenchymal chondrosarcoma: An

immunohistochemical study. Ann Diagn Pathol 2021;50:151660.

78. Hornick JL, Fletcher CD. Myoepithelial tumors of soft tissue: a clinicopathologic and immunohisto-chemical study of 101 cases with evaluation of prognostic parameters. Am J Surg Pathol 2003; 27:1183–96.

79. Antonescu CR, Zhang L, Chang NE, et al. EWSR1-POU5F1 fusion in soft tissue myoepithelial tumors. A molecular analysis of sixty-six cases, including soft tissue, bone, and visceral lesions, showing common involvement of the EWSR1 gene. Genes Chromosomes Cancer 2010;49:1114–24.

80. Bridge JA, Sumegi J, Druta M, et al. Clinical, pathological, and genomic features of EWSR1-PATZ1 fusion sarcoma. Mod Pathol 2019;32:1593–604.

81. Michal M, Rubin BP, Agaimy A, et al. EWSR1-PATZ1-rearranged sarcoma: a report of nine cases of spindle and round cell neoplasms with predilection for thoracoabdominal soft tissues and frequent expression of neural and skeletal muscle markers. Mod Pathol 2021;34:770–85.

82. Dembla V, Somaiah N, Barata P, et al. Prevalence of MDM2 amplification and co-alterations in 523 advanced cancer patients in the MD Anderson phase 1 clinic. Oncotarget 2018;9:33232–43.

83. Park KW, Cai Y, Benjamin T, et al. Round Cell Sarcoma with EWSR1-PATZ1 Gene Fusion in the Neck: Case Report and Review of the Literature. Laryngoscope 2020;130:E833–6.

84. Yau DTW, Wong S, Chow C, et al. Round Cell Sarcoma with EWSR1-PATZ1 Fusion in the Face of a Five-Year-Old Boy: Report of a Case with Unusual Histologic Features. Head Neck Pathol 2021;15:1350–8.

85. Ngo C, Khneisser P, Kanaan C, et al. Sarcome avec transcrit de fusion EWSR1-PATZ1 - Une nouvelle observation avec revue de la littérature [EWSR1-PATZ1 fusion sarcoma - A new case report and review of the literature]. Ann Pathol 2021;41:207–11.

86. Mastrangelo T, Modena P, Tornielli S, et al. A novel zinc finger gene is fused to EWS in small round cell tumor. Oncogene 2000;19:3799–804.

87. Chougule A, Taylor MS, Nardi V, et al. Spindle and Round Cell Sarcoma With EWSR1-PATZ1 Gene Fusion: A Sarcoma With Polyphenotypic Differentiation. Am J Surg Pathol 2019;43:220–8.

88. Mito JK, Qian X, Doyle LA, et al. Role of Histone H3K27 Trimethylation Loss as a Marker for Malignant Peripheral Nerve Sheath Tumor in Fine-Needle Aspiration and Small Biopsy Specimens. Am J Clin Pathol 2017;148:179–89.

89. Miettinen MM, Antonescu CR, Fletcher CDM, et al. Histopathologic evaluation of atypical neurofibromatous tumors and their transformation into malignant peripheral nerve sheath tumor in patients with neurofibromatosis 1-a consensus overview. Hum Pathol 2017;67:1–10.

90. Mazuelas H, Uriarte-Arrazola I, Negro A, et al. Deep genomic analysis of malignant peripheral nerve sheath tumor cell lines challenges current malignant peripheral nerve sheath tumor diagnosis. iScience 2023;26:106096.

91. Benini S, Gamberi G, Cocchi S, et al. Identification of a novel fusion transcript EWSR1-VEZF1 by anchored multiplex PCR in malignant peripheral nerve sheath tumor. Pathol Res Pract 2020;216:152760.

92. Chan JA, McMenamin ME, Fletcher CD. Synovial sarcoma in older patients: clinicopathological analysis of 32 cases with emphasis on unusual histological features. Histopathology 2003;43:72–83.

93. Baranov E, McBride MJ, Bellizzi AM, et al. A Novel SS18-SSX Fusion-specific Antibody for the Diagnosis of Synovial Sarcoma. Am J Surg Pathol 2020;44:922–33.

94. Suurmeijer AJH, Song W, Sung YS, et al. Novel recurrent PHF1-TFE3 fusions in ossifying fibromyxoid tumors. Genes Chromosomes Cancer 2019;58:643–9.

95. Gebre-Medhin S, Nord KH, Möller E, et al. Recurrent rearrangement of the PHF1 gene in ossifying fibromyxoid tumors. Am J Pathol 2012;181:1069–77.

96. Doyle LA, Vivero M, Fletcher CD, et al. Nuclear expression of STAT6 distinguishes solitary fibrous tumor from histologic mimics. Mod Pathol 2014;27:390–5.

97. Baranov E, Hornick JL. Soft Tissue Special Issue: Fibroblastic and Myofibroblastic Neoplasms of the Head and Neck. Head Neck Pathol 2020;14:43–58.

98. Bianchi G, Sambri A, Pedrini E, et al. Histological and molecular features of solitary fibrous tumor of the extremities: clinical correlation. Virchows Arch 2020;476:445–54.

99. Antonescu CR, Agaram NP, Sung YS, et al. A Distinct Malignant Epithelioid Neoplasm With GLI1 Gene Rearrangements, Frequent S100 Protein Expression, and Metastatic Potential: Expanding the Spectrum of Pathologic Entities With ACTB/MALAT1/PTCH1-GLI1 Fusions. Am J Surg Pathol 2018;42:553–60.

100. Agaram NP, Zhang L, Sung YS, et al. GLI1-amplifications expand the spectrum of soft tissue neoplasms defined by GLI1 gene fusions. Mod Pathol 2019;32:1617–26.

101. Parrack PH, Mariño-Enríquez A, Fletcher CDM, et al. GLI1 Immunohistochemistry Distinguishes Mesenchymal Neoplasms With GLI1 Alterations From Morphologic Mimics. Am J Surg Pathol 2023;47:453–60.

102. Jo VY, Mariño-Enríquez A, Fletcher CD. Epithelioid rhabdomyosarcoma: clinicopathologic analysis of 16 cases of a morphologically distinct variant of rhabdomyosarcoma. Am J Surg Pathol 2011;35:1523–30.

103. Xu B, Suurmeijer AJH, Agaram NP, et al. Head and neck rhabdomyosarcoma with TFCP2 fusions and ALK overexpression: a clinicopathological and molecular analysis of 11 cases. Histopathology 2021;79: 347–57.

104. Rutland CD, Gedallovich J, Wang A, et al. Diagnostic utility of FOXO1 immunohistochemistry for rhabdomyosarcoma classification. Histopathology 2023;83(1):49–56.

105. Agaram NP, Zhang L, Sung YS, et al. Expanding the Spectrum of Intraosseous Rhabdomyosarcoma: Correlation Between 2 Distinct Gene Fusions and Phenotype. Am J Surg Pathol 2019;43: 695–702.

Xanthogranulomatous Epithelial Tumors and Keratin-Positive Giant Cell Rich Tumors of Soft Tissue and Bone
Two Sides of the Same Coin

Andrew L. Folpe, MD

KEYWORDS

- Xanthogranulomatous epithelial tumor • Keratin-positive giant cell-rich tumor • HMGA2 • NCOR2
- Immunohistochemistry • Molecular genetics

Key points

- Xanthogranulomatous epithelial tumors are extremely rare and occur in both soft tissue and bone.
- Histopathologic features include xanthomatous histiocytes, osteoclast-like giant cells, and difficult-to-identify epithelioid mononuclear cells, sometimes with eosinophilic cytoplasm.
- Keratin immunostains highlight the diagnostic epithelioid cells.
- Targeted molecular genetic study often identifies *HMGA2::NCOR2* in xanthogranulomatous epithelial tumors.

ABSTRACT

Xanthogranulomatous epithelial tumor is a recently described soft tissue tumor characterized by subcutaneous location, partial encapsulation, a xanthogranulomatous inflammatory cell infiltrate, and keratin-positive mononuclear cells. It shares some morphologic features with keratin-positive, giant cell-rich soft tissue tumors. Both have recently been shown to harbor HMGA2::NCOR2 fusions. The relationship between these tumors and their differential diagnosis with other osteoclast-containing soft tissue tumors is discussed.

OVERVIEW

Xanthogranulomatous epithelial tumor (XGET), first described by Fritchie and colleagues[1] in 2020, is a very rare, low-grade mesenchymal tumor occurring in both soft tissue and osseous locations, with a strong female predilection. Shortly thereafter, two series of keratin-positive, giant cell-rich tumors of soft tissue and bone harboring *HMGA2::NCOR2* fusions were reported by Agaimy and colleagues[2] and Panagopoulos and colleagues,[3] respectively. Most recently, Dehner and colleagues[4] studied 9 tumors showing overlapping morphologic features of XGET and keratin-positive, giant cell-rich tumor, demonstrating *HMGA2::NCOR2* fusions in 7. The overlapping morphologic, immunohistochemical, and molecular genetic features of XGET and keratin-positive, giant cell-rich tumor strongly suggest that these represent somewhat different morphologic manifestations of a single entity, and they will be discussed together.

CLINICAL FEATURES

Inclusive of these 4 series, 26 cases of xanthogranulomatous epithelial tumor/keratin-positive, giant cell-rich tumor have been reported. One fusion-

---

Department of Pathology and Laboratory Medicine, Mayo Clinic, Rochester, MN 55905, USA
E-mail address: folpe.andrew@mayo.edu

Surgical Pathology 17 (2024) 57–64
https://doi.org/10.1016/j.path.2023.07.002
1875-9181/24/© 2023 Elsevier Inc. All rights reserved.

negative tumor from the Dehner and colleagues series (case 7) has subsequently been shown to represent a chondroblastoma (Dr. Carina Dehner, personal communication, 2023).

The tumors are far more common in women (20 women; 6 men) and generally occur in young adults, with median ages of 21-33 years in these 4 series. Exceptional cases have been reported in children and in elderly patients. In the soft tissues, the tumors present as subcutaneous masses of variable size, without a clear site predisposition (**Fig. 1**A). Similarly, osseous tumors may involve either the axial or appendicular skeleton. Radiographically, osseous tumors typically appear as mixed lytic and sclerotic lesions with a soft tissue component.[1]

Clinical follow-up has been reported for 17 patients with xanthogranulomatous epithelial tumor/keratin-positive, giant cell-rich tumor; all are reported to be disease-free, without local recurrences or metastases. I have, however, seen in consultation a xanthogranulomatous epithelial tumor of a cervical vertebra which recurred locally roughly 2 years after initial presentation.

PATHOLOGICAL FEATURES

Xanthogranulomatous epithelial tumors present as uninodular masses, often surrounded at least in part by a fibrous pseudocapsule. They tend to be dominated by sheets of foamy macrophages, Touton-type multinucleated giant cells, a mixed inflammatory cell infiltrate, and a variable number of osteoclast-like giant cells; cholesterol clefts and small foci of necrosis may also be present (**Fig. 1**B–D). Careful inspection, however, discloses small aggregates of cytologically atypical epithelioid cells, sometimes with distinctly eosinophilic, vaguely squamoid cytoplasm (**Fig. 2**). These epithelioid cells are positive with broad-spectrum keratin antibodies (eg, OSCAR and AE1/AE3) and occasionally for high-molecular-weight keratins.[1,4]

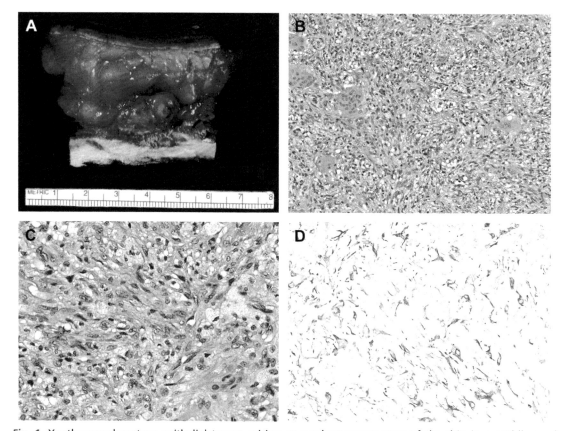

Fig. 1. Xanthogranulomatous epithelial tumor, arising as a subcutaneous mass of the shin in a middle-aged woman, with invasion of the underlying tibia (A). The tumor was composed of an admixture of osteoclast-like giant cells, lipid-laden macrophages, smaller non-lipidized macrophages and other mononuclear cells (B). Higher power magnification, showing scattered mononuclear cells with enlarged, irregular nuclei (C). A keratin AE1/AE3 immunostain was positive in the mononuclear cells, highlighting dendritic processes inapparent on the routinely stained slide (D).

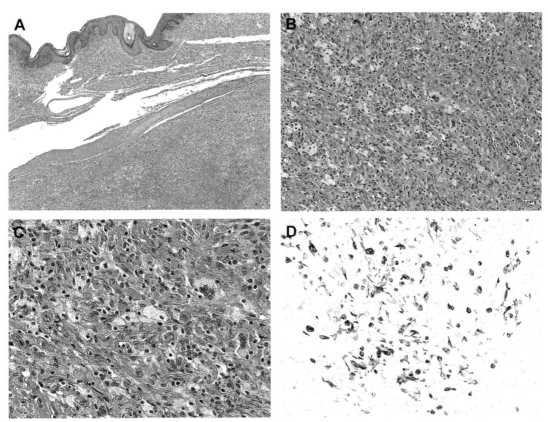

Fig. 2. Xanthogranulomatous epithelial tumor, presenting as a well-circumscribed, partially encapsulated mass in the subcutis of the thigh in a middle-aged woman (*A*). Numerous lipidized macrophages and occasional Touton-type giant cells are present (*B*). At higher power magnification, scattered mononuclear cells with brightly eosinophilic cytoplasm are seen (*C*). These cells were keratin-positive (*D*). This tumor was found to harbor *HMGA2::NCOR2* by next-generation sequencing.

Endothelial and myoid markers are negative; SMARCB1 expression and SMARCA4 expression are retained (normal). Those tumors previously reported as "keratin-positive, giant cell-rich tumors" lack xanthomatous cells and Touton-type giant cells, and consist largely of bland epithelioid to spindled mononuclear cells admixed with large numbers of osteoclast-like giant cells[2] (**Fig. 3**). Occasional cases show overlapping morphologic features, such that the distinction between xanthogranulomatous epithelial tumor and keratin-positive, giant cell-rich tumor may be arbitrary.[4] Importantly, both XGET and keratin-positive, giant cell-rich tumors present as single nodules, unlike the distinctive, multinodular, vaguely plexiform growth pattern which characterizes soft tissue giant cell tumors (see later in discussion for additional discussion).

GENETIC FEATURES

HMGA2::NCOR2 fusions have been reported in 18 xanthogranulomatous epithelial tumors/keratin-positive, giant cell-rich tumors, most often involving exon 3 of *HMGA2* and exon 16 of *NCOR2*.[1–4] It is difficult to estimate the actual frequency of this genetic event in these tumors, as for example only fusion-positive tumors were reported by Panagopoulos and colleagues,[3] whereas Fritchie and colleagues[1] did not identify any fusion events in cases studied at Mayo Clinic with next-generation sequencing. We have recently re-evaluated some of our previous sequencing data, and found a small number of reads in some cases, with positive results for *HMGA2::NCOR2* by targeted reverse transcriptase polymerase chain reaction (Dr. Ying-Chun Lo, Mayo Clinic, Rochester MN, unpublished observations, 2023). This suggests that *HMGA2::NCOR2* fusions may eventually be identified in most, if not all, xanthogranulomatous epithelial tumor/keratin-positive, giant cell-rich tumors.

DIFFERENTIAL DIAGNOSIS

The differential diagnosis for xanthogranulomatous epithelial tumor/keratin-positive, giant cell-

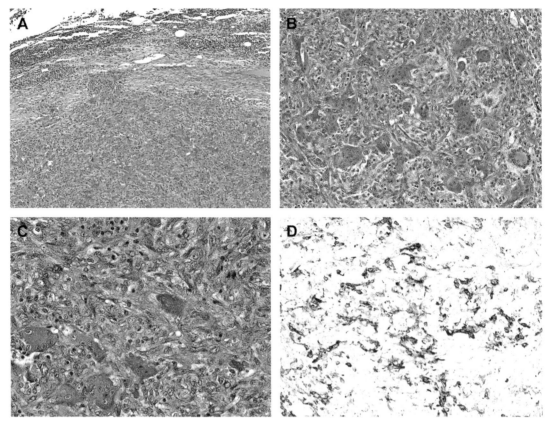

Fig. 3. In contrast to soft tissue giant cell tumors, which are unencapsulated, multinodular, and dermal-based, xanthogranulomatous epithelial tumors present as uninodular, partially encapsulated masses in the subcutis (*A*). Some xanthogranulomatous epithelial tumors may contain large numbers of osteoclast-like giant cells, mimicking soft tissue giant cell tumor (*B*). The intervening mononuclear cells have slightly enlarged, irregular nuclei (*C*). As expected, these mononuclear cells are keratin-positive, again showing somewhat dendritic morphology (*D*). This case was found to be *HMGA2::NCOR2*-positive.

rich tumor centers on other osteoclast-rich tumors of soft tissue and bone, including giant cell tumor of bone (**Fig. 4**A, B), soft tissue giant cell tumor (**Fig. 4**C–F), osteoclast-rich undifferentiated pleomorphic sarcoma (so-called malignant giant cell tumor of soft parts) (**Fig. 5**A, B), other osteoclast-rich malignancies (eg, carcinoma, melanoma) (**Fig. 5**C, D), solitary (juvenile) xanthogranuloma (**Fig. 5**E, F), and tenosynovial giant cell tumor (**Fig. 6**).

Giant cell tumors of bone usually consist of sheets of osteoclast-like giant cells and bland mononuclear cells, typically lack xanthogranulomatous features, harbor mutations in *H3F3A* at the Gly34 codon, and express histone 3 G34W (H3G34W) immunohistochemically. Soft tissue giant cell tumors usually present in the dermis and subcutis as multiple small nodules, sometimes with a peripheral shell of bone, and lack H3G34W expression. This multinodular growth pattern is highly characteristic of soft tissue giant cell tumors, and helps to distinguish them from keratin-positive, giant cell-rich soft tumors.

Osteoclast-rich undifferentiated pleomorphic sarcomas typically present as larger masses, often with large areas of necrosis, and contain mononuclear cells with overt cytologic atypia, unlike the generally bland cells seen in xanthogranulomatous epithelial tumor/keratin-positive, giant cell-rich tumor (see **Fig. 5**A, B). Similarly, although osteoclast-rich carcinomas share keratin expression with xanthogranulomatous epithelial tumor/keratin-positive, giant cell-rich tumor, they would not be expected to present as encapsulated subcutaneous masses (see **Fig. 5**C, D). Immunohistochemistry for melanoma-associated markers (eg, S100 protein, HMB45) should allow for confident diagnosis of melanomas containing osteoclast-like giant cells.

Solitary xanthogranulomas almost always involve the skin, and consist of bland histiocytoid cells with

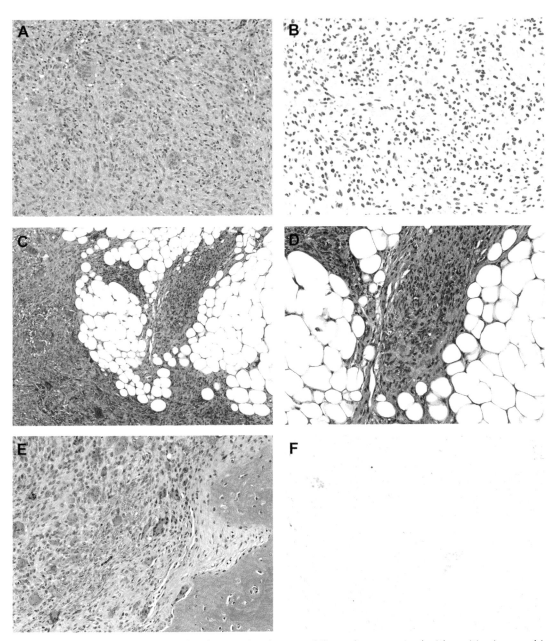

Fig. 4. Giant cell tumors of bone with soft tissue involvement (*A*) may be recognized with positive immunohistochemistry for histone G34W (*B*). Soft tissue giant cell tumors grow as multiple minute nodules in the dermis and subcutis, unlike xanthogranulomatous epithelial tumors (*C*). Higher power view of a minute nodule of soft tissue giant cell tumor (*D*). Metaplastic bone formation is often seen (*E*). Despite being morphologically identical to giant cell tumors of bone, soft tissue giant cell tumors lack histone G34W expression (*F*).

folded or grooved nuclei displaying a variable degree of cytoplasmic lipid accumulation, chronic inflammatory cells including eosinophils, and sometimes Touton-type giant cells. Keratin expression is absent, with the lesional cells themselves usually co-expressing Factor 13a and markers of histiocytic lineage, such as CD163 and CD11c.

Tenosynovial giant cell tumors, neoplasms of (usually) *CSF1*-rearanged synoviocytes, are composed of an admixture of small histiocytes, larger eosinophilic synoviocytes (often containing a ring of intracytoplasmic iron), chronic inflammatory cells, foamy macrophages, and osteoclast-like giant cells. The relative number of osteoclast-like giant

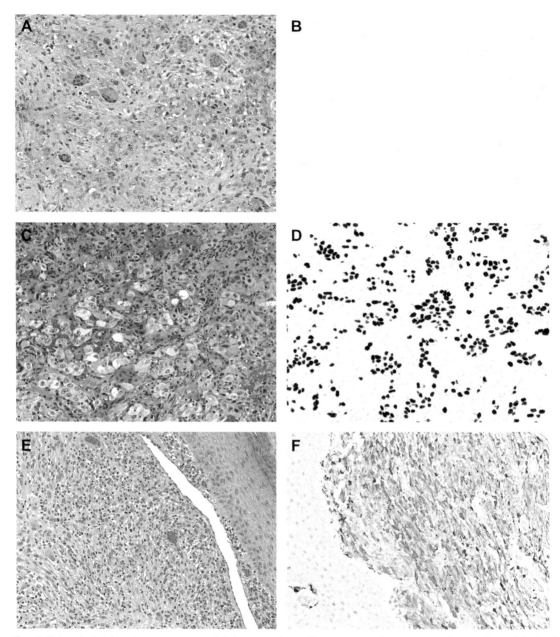

Fig. 5. Osteoclast-rich osteosarcoma, containing overtly malignant-appearing mononuclear cells and foci of osteoid production (*A*). Negative immunohistochemistry for histone G34W helps to distinguish this form of osteosarcoma from malignant giant cell tumor of bone (*B*). Not all osteoclast-rich, keratin-positive tumors of soft tissue are xanthogranulomatous epithelial tumors. This subcutaneous nodule (*C*) presented in an adult male with a history of pulmonary adenocarcinoma and was strongly positive for TTF1 (*D*) and napsin (not shown). Unlike xanthogranulomatous epithelial tumor, solitary (juvenile) xanthogranuloma tends to involve the skin and often contains numerous eosinophils (*E*). Co-expression of Factor XIIIa (*F*) and histiocytic markers such as CD163 characterize solitary xanthogranuloma.

cells, small histiocytes, and foamy macrophages is highly variable, and many tenosynovial giant cell tumors lack giant cells altogether. Other useful clues to the diagnosis of tenosynovial giant cell tumor include "zonation," with the peripheral accumulation of foamy macrophages, abundant hyalinized collagen, and pseudoalveolar spaces. Synoviocytes express clusterin, CSF1 mRNA and sometimes desmin by immunohistochemistry, and are keratin-negative. Morphologically, synoviocytes

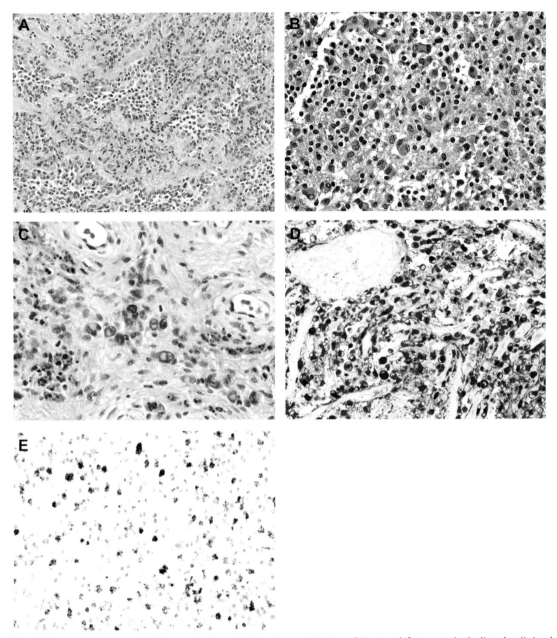

Fig. 6. Tenosynovial giant cell tumors often display characteristic architectural features, including hyalinized collagen and pseudoalveolar spaces (*A*). Despite their name, these are neoplasms of synoviocytes, the large, eosinophilic mononuclear cells seen here, and often lack appreciable numbers of osteoclasts (*B*). Intracytoplasmic iron pigment is often present in synoviocytes (*C*). In challenging cases, immunohistochemistry for clusterin (*D*) and in-situ hybridization for CSF1 mRNA (*E*) can help to identify synoviocytes.

appear as relatively large histiocytoid cells with eosinophilic cytoplasm and a characteristic ring of intracytoplasmic iron. None of the tumors in the differential diagnosis of xanthogranulomatous epithelial tumor/keratin-positive, giant cell-rich tumor would be expected to harbor *HMGA2::NCOR2* fusions, of course.

CLINICS CARE POINTS

- Unlike soft tissue giant cell tumors, xanthogranulomatous epithelial tumors lack metaplastic bone and contain keratin-positive cells.

- Solitary xanthogranulomas also lack keratin-positive cells and are composed of bland spindled to histiocytoid cells showing diffuse Factor 13A expression.

- The presence of mononuclear cells with high nuclear grade should point towards giant cell-rich osteosarcoma, undifferentiated sarcoma, carcinoma, or melanoma.

- Tenosynovial giant cell tumors are neoplasms of clusterin- and CSF1 mRNA-positive synoviocytes, lacking keratin expression.

REFERENCES

1. Fritchie KJ, Torres-Mora J, Inwards C, et al. Xanthogranulomatous epithelial tumor: report of 6 cases of a novel, potentially deceptive lesion with a predilection for young women. Mod Pathol 2020;33(10):1889–95.

2. Agaimy A, Michal M, Stoehr R, et al. Recurrent novel HMGA2-NCOR2 fusions characterize a subset of keratin-positive giant cell-rich soft tissue tumors. Mod Pathol 2021;34(8):1507–20.

3. Panagopoulos I, Andersen K, Gorunova L, et al. Recurrent fusion of the genes for high-mobility group AT-hook 2 (HMGA2) and nuclear receptor co-repressor 2 (NCOR2) in osteoclastic giant cell-rich tumors of bone. Cancer Genomics Proteomics 2022; 19(2):163–77.

4. Dehner CA, Baker JC, Bell R, et al. Xanthogranulomatous epithelial tumors and keratin-positive giant cell-rich soft tissue tumors: two aspects of a single entity with frequent HMGA2-NCOR2 fusions. Mod Pathol 2022;35(11):1656–66.

Inflammatory Rhabdomyoblastic Tumor
From a Nebulous Smooth Muscle Neoplasm to a Novel Skeletal Muscle Tumor Subtype

Michael Michal, MD, PhD[a,b,]*

KEYWORDS

- Inflammatory rhabdomyoblastic tumor • Inflammatory leiomyosarcoma • Rhabdomyosarcoma
- Skeletal muscle tumor • Near haploidization

Key points

- Inflammatory rhabdomyoblastic tumor (IRMT) is a recently introduced name for tumors currently included in the World Health Organization classification of soft tissue tumors under the rubric inflammatory leiomyosarcoma.
- The suggested nomenclature change is based on recently presented morphologic, immunohistochemical, and gene expression profiling evidence of skeletal muscle differentiation in these neoplasms.
- Although most cases follow an indolent clinical course, a subset of IRMT may progress to rhabdomyosarcoma.
- IRMT is a morphologically distinctive soft tissue tumor characterized by a mostly well-circumscribed growth; dense chronic inflammatory infiltrate; aggregates of xanthoma cells; and scattered, often pleomorphic tumor cells with minimal mitotic activity.
- On a cytogenetic level, most cases show a virtually diagnostic near-haploid karyotype with retained biparental disomy of chromosomes 5 and 22 with or without subsequent whole genome doubling.

ABSTRACT

Inflammatory rhabdomyoblastic tumor is a recently introduced name for neoplasms currently included in the World Health Organization classification of soft tissue tumors under the rubric inflammatory leiomyosarcoma. Inflammatory rhabdomyoblastic tumor is an excellent example of how surgical pathologists working in conjunction with tumor biologists can greatly improve tumor classification to the benefit of patients. Over the last 28 years, understanding of this entity has undergone a fascinating evolution. This review serves as a summary of the latest findings in inflammatory rhabdomyoblastic tumor research and a diagnostic manual for the practicing surgical pathologist.

HISTORICAL PERSPECTIVE

Inflammatory rhabdomyoblastic tumor (IRMT) is a recently introduced name for a mostly indolent and morphologically distinctive soft tissue tumor characterized by a dense chronic inflammatory infiltrate, aggregates of xanthoma cells, and scattered, often pleomorphic tumor cells with morphologic, immunohistochemical, and gene expression

[a] Department of Pathology, Charles University, Faculty of Medicine in Plzen, Czech Republic; [b] Bioptical Laboratory, Ltd, Plzen, Czech Republic
* Corresponding author. Department of Pathology, Charles University, Medical Faculty and Charles University Hospital Plzen, Alej Svobody 80, 323 00, Plzen.
E-mail address: michael.michal@biopticka.cz

Surgical Pathology 17 (2024) 65–76
https://doi.org/10.1016/j.path.2023.06.008
1875-9181/24/© 2023 Elsevier Inc. All rights reserved.

profiling evidence of skeletal muscle differentiation. On a cytogenetic level, most cases show a virtually diagnostic near-haploid karyotype with retained biparental disomy of chromosomes 5 and 22 with or without subsequent whole genome doubling.[1,2]

Over the last 28 years, the understanding of this entity has undergone a fascinating evolution. The story began in 1995 when Merchant and colleagues[3] published a series of 12 tumors with morphologic and immunohistochemical features reminiscent of smooth muscle differentiation admixed with a prominent inflammatory component, mainly in the form of aggregates of xanthoma cells and lymphocytes, that had previously fallen within the category of inflammatory malignant fibrous histiocytoma. Based on the cytomorphologic features, coupled with the immunohistochemical expression of desmin, muscle specific actin, and smooth muscle actin by some of the neoplastic cells, these tumors were thought to represent a smooth muscle neoplasm and the term inflammatory leiomyosarcoma (ILMS) was coined. Three years later, the first cytogenetic analysis of ILMS revealed a highly unusual and characteristic chromosomal pattern consisting of a near-haploid genome.[4] Apart from these two studies, only a small case series and scattered case reports had been published on this topic over the span of the subsequent 20 years.[5–7] The revived interest in this topic dates to 2017 when Arbajian and colleagues[8] reported a thorough molecular study of ILMS that, apart from confirming the clearly nonrandom and characteristic pattern of near-haploid genome, revealed several novel findings. Most importantly, their gene expression profiling data showed upregulation of genes, such as MYOD1, MYOG, PAX7, MYF5, and MYF6, all of which are known to be crucial for skeletal muscle development and their expression in normal tissues is fairly restricted to skeletal muscle. However, they did not confirm the overexpression of proteins encoded by these genes using immunohistochemistry. A year later, Martinez and colleagues[9] reported what was thought to be a novel group of neoplasms called histiocyte-rich rhabdomyoblastic tumor (HRRMT). Because this article was published at a time when our group was working on another study on ILMS, we noticed their cohort of HRRMT showed clinical, morphologic, and immunohistochemical features virtually identical to ours, but in addition was shown to consistently express skeletal muscle markers. The results of studies by Arbajian and Martinez led us to analyze the expression of MyoD1, myogenin, and PAX7 (ie, the three most widely used skeletal muscle markers) on our cohort of ILMS and, unsurprisingly, most cases in our study showed positive expression. Based on these overlapping findings, we suggested in our study that ILMS and so-called HRRMT represent the same entities.[10] However, at that time, we were not able to confirm the presence of the near-haploid genome in our cases, which was the last necessary step to prove our assumption. This final step was done by Cloutier and colleagues[1] in their 2020 article where they studied cases previously reported as both ILMS and HRRMT. They confirmed the presence of the same near-haploid genome, and all other overlapping clinicopathologic features in both groups. They also proposed the term IRMT which, as arguably the most fitting one, will likely be adopted as the official name in the next World Health Organization classification instead of the ILMS terminology used in the current edition.

Another milestone were the recent findings that a small subset of IRMT may serve as a precursor lesion for the development of high-grade rhabdomyosarcoma (RMS).[2,11,12] Although such cases of RMS arising from IRMT are apparently rare (estimated as 6 out of >200 analyzed cases of RMS in the study by Dehner and colleagues[2]), their existence represents an important caveat in IRMT diagnosis. They also represent an interesting conceptual shift in RMS pathogenesis, because RMS was thought to always arise de novo. Nevertheless, a small subset of RMS may apparently arise from a precursor lesion, such as IRMT,[2] or as other recently published studies have shown, from biphenotypic sinonasal sarcoma.[13–15]

In addition, there remains a small group of lesions with an apparent predilection for pulmonary origin, which morphologically overlap with IRMT, but lack the near-haploid genetic background. Moreover, apart from consistent desmin and occasional smooth muscle actin expression, they lack a well-defined smooth or skeletal muscle immunophenotype. Although the term "low-grade inflammatory myoid tumor" was suggested, the terminology for these poorly understood tumors remains to be solidified and their relationship to IRMT awaits further investigation.[16]

CLINICAL FEATURES

IRMT typically presents as a slow-growing deeply located intramuscular lesion with a predilection for the extremities, particularly the thigh, followed by the back/paravertebral locations and cervical soft tissues (Table 1). Rare cases may arise in the retroperitoneum,[10] sometimes originating from the retroperitoneal portion of the psoas muscle (unpublished observation). They preferentially occur

Table 1
Key clinical features

Age	Median ~40 y (range, 17–69 y)
Male/female ratio	Distinct male predilection
Size	Median ~4 cm (range, 2.1–11.5 cm)
Location	Intramuscular lesion on the extremities (thigh) > back/paravertebral > neck; rarely elsewhere (retroperitoneum)
Clinical behavior	Mostly indolent tumors A subset may progress to rhabdomyosarcoma
Association with tumor syndromes	Occasional association with NF1, one patient with Lynch syndrome

in male patients with a median age at diagnosis around 40 years (range, 17–69 years) with a median size around 4 cm (range, 2.1–11.5 cm).[1,8,10,12,17,18] Association with type 1 neurofibromatosis has been occasionally reported[1,18] and one case occurred in a patient with hereditary nonpolyposis colorectal cancer syndrome.[12]

Conventional IRMT are indolent tumors that, when completely excised, usually do not recur or metastasize.[1,10,12,18] Only individual cases of conventional IRMT with recurrence or metastasis have been reported but mostly in older literature where the diagnosis is uncertain.[3,5,10] However, recent reports have shown that a small subset of IRMT may progress to RMS and follow an aggressive clinical course. Such cases have similar clinical features as the conventional ones, but they seem to affect slightly older patients (median, 50 years).[2]

Out of seven reported cases, one recurred and six metastasized. The patients from the latter group were treated with a variable combination of surgery, radiotherapy, and/or chemotherapy and one patient died of disease and the others were alive with disease.[2,12]

PATHOLOGIC FEATURES

A prototypical example of IRMT presents as a well-circumscribed and partially encapsulated intramuscular mass (**Fig. 1**, **Table 2**) with occasional small foci of infiltration into the surrounding soft tissues. Hemosiderin deposition, scattered intralesional calcifications (**Fig. 2**), and lymphoid aggregates located particularly around the tumor capsule are common. One of the hallmarks of the tumor are interspersed lymphocytes, plasma cells, and Touton-type giant cells, along with large aggregates of xanthoma cells (**Figs. 1** and **2**) and inconspicuous but widespread spindled histiocytes admixed in between the neoplastic cells (**Fig. 3**). Other inflammatory cell types, such as eosinophils and especially neutrophils, are less prominent. The neoplastic cells are arranged haphazardly or in short fascicles (**Fig. 1**) and consist of a pleomorphic mixture of spindled, epithelioid to rhabdoid cells (lacking cross-striations) with abundant eosinophilic cytoplasm (**Fig. 3**). Some of the neoplastic cells may show bizarre, angulated cell shapes (**Fig. 4A**). Marked regional variation in the appearance of the neoplastic cells may be observed within one tumor. Although some areas may contain abundant epithelioid to rhabdoid cells (**Fig. 5A**) others may be almost purely spindled (**Fig. 5B**). Nuclear pleomorphism and hyperchromatism are common (**Fig. 3**) and multilobated nuclei may be present (**Fig. 4A**).[1,2,10] In contrast to the atypical

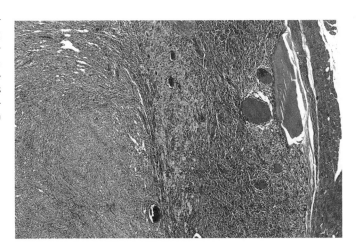

Fig. 1. A prototypical example of IRMT presents as a well-circumscribed and partially encapsulated intramuscular mass. Occasional small foci of infiltration into the surrounding soft tissues may be present (not shown). The neoplastic cells are arranged haphazardly or in short fascicles and are frequently admixed with large aggregates of xanthoma cells.

Table 2
Morphologic key features

Border	Well-circumscribed, often with pseudocapsule, small areas with infiltration
Architecture	Fascicular to haphazard
Neoplastic cell appearance	Pleomorphic mixture of spindled, epithelioid to rhabdoid cells (lacking cross-striations) with abundant eosinophilic cytoplasm Some neoplastic cells may show bizarre, angulated cell shapes Nuclear pleomorphism and hyperchromatism common
Inflammatory cells	Dispersed lymphocytes and plasma cells Diffusely admixed spindled histiocytes and histiocytic aggregates Lymphoid aggregates around pseudocapsule
Mitotic activity	Extremely low in most cases (<1/10 high-powered field)
Necrosis	Usually absent, focal if present
Morphologic signs of rhabdomyosarcomatous progression	Two patterns of progression: 1. Gradual transition to foci with fewer inflammatory cells and predominance of monotonous, epithelioid to rhabdoid neoplastic cells with low mitotic rate 2. Highly cellular proliferation of spindled to epithelioid cells with marked nuclear atypia, frequent mitotic figures, and coagulative tumor necrosis

cytomorphology, mitotic activity is usually disproportionately low, because most cases have less than or equal to one mitotic figure per 10 high-power fields[1,10,19] (**Fig. 3**) and only occasional cases show two to three mitotic figures per 10 high-power fields.[8,10] Similarly, using the Ki-67 (Mib-1) antibody, the proliferative indices usually range from 1% to 5%.[10] Small foci with necrosis may rarely be found but extensive necrotic areas are absent.[10,18,19]

In cases where IRMT progresses to RMS, the morphologic changes may show two distinct patterns, which are found in primary tumors and in metastases. As described by Dehner and colleagues,[2] the first recognizable form of tumor progression in IRMT consists of a gradual transition

from areas of typical IRMT, with abundant lymphohistiocytic infiltrate containing only scattered neoplastic cells with often bizarre cell appearance (see **Fig. 4**A), to foci where the inflammatory cell infiltrate is less prominent, and rhabdomyoblastic tumor cells are arranged in aggregates of varying sizes. Paradoxically, the neoplastic cells in these areas are often much less bizarre-appearing than in typical IRMT and consist instead of rather small, monotonous, epithelioid to rhabdoid cells with a modest amount of eosinophilic cytoplasm, evenly dispersed chromatin, small nucleoli, and a low mitotic rate (see **Fig. 4**B). This pattern of progression in IRMT may be seen by itself or in combination with further morphologic progression in the form of a highly cellular proliferation of spindled

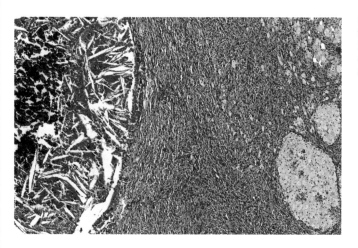

Fig. 2. Hallmarks of the tumor include frequent intralesional calcifications, interspersed lymphocytes and plasma cells, and larger aggregates of xanthoma cells.

Fig. 3. The neoplastic cells consist of a pleomorphic mixture of spindled, epithelioid to rhabdoid cells (lacking cross-striations) with abundant eosinophilic cytoplasm. Nuclear pleomorphism and hyperchromatism are common. The diffusely present spindled histiocytes admixed in between the neoplastic cells are not readily identifiable on hematoxylin-eosin stain. In contrast to the atypical morphology of the neoplastic cells, mitotic activity is usually disproportionately low, and most cases have less than or equal to one mitotic figure per 10 high-power fields.

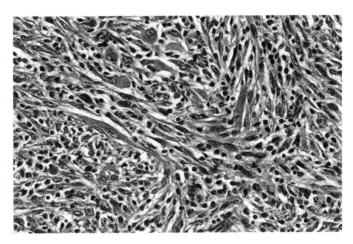

to epithelioid cells with marked nuclear atypia, frequent mitotic figures including atypical forms, and coagulative tumor necrosis. Morphologic evidence of skeletal muscle differentiation is not obvious in this second pattern (**Fig. 4**C), and immunohistochemistry for skeletal muscle markers is necessary for definite classification as RMS.[2]

IMMUNOHISTOCHEMICAL FEATURES

IRMT has a skeletal muscle immunophenotype with typically diffuse expression of desmin (**Fig. 6**) and more limited expression of MyoD1, PAX7, and myogenin (**Table 3**). Of the latter three, PAX7 tends to show the most extensive expression, whereas MyoD1 and especially myogenin often show focal

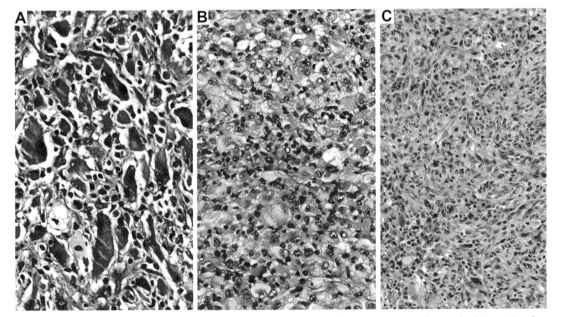

Fig. 4. The progression of IRMT into RMS may show two patterns. The first consists of a gradual transition from areas of typical IRMT, with abundant lymphohistiocytic infiltrate containing only scattered neoplastic cells with often bizarre cell appearance (*A*), to foci where the inflammatory cell infiltrate is less prominent, and the neoplastic cells in these areas are often much less bizarre-appearing than in typical IRMT and consist instead of rather small, monotonous, epithelioid to rhabdoid cells with a modest amount of eosinophilic cytoplasm, evenly dispersed chromatin, small nucleoli, and a low mitotic rate (*B*). The second pattern (*C*) consists of a highly cellular proliferation of spindled to epithelioid cells with marked nuclear atypia, frequent mitotic figures including atypical forms, and coagulative tumor necrosis (not shown). Morphologic evidence of skeletal muscle differentiation is not obvious in this second pattern. (*Photomicrographs Courtesy of* A.L. Folpe, MD, Rochester, MN.)

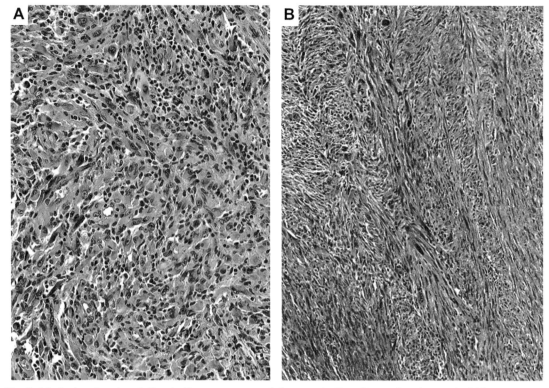

Fig. 5. Marked regional variation in the appearance of the neoplastic cells may be observed within one tumor. Although some areas may contain abundant epithelioid to rhabdoid cells (*A*), others may be almost purely spindled (*B*).

expression (**Fig. 7**A-C). Occasional cases may be negative with some of these markers, most often myogenin.[1,10] Some desmin-positive cells show a histiocyte-like foamy cytoplasm, which is a useful diagnostic clue (see **Fig. 6**).[10] CD163 stains the aggregates of xanthoma cells and the remarkably high number of spindled histiocytes diffusely admixed among the CD163-negative and desmin-positive neoplastic cells (**Fig. 7**D), a feature not readily identifiable on hematoxylin-eosin stain. Many cases also show variable smooth muscle actin

expression.[1,10] Although former studies (including ours) reported positivity with a nonspecific h-caldesmon antibody clone (E89),[8,10] using the smooth muscle-specific h-CD clone, h-caldesmon is negative in IRMT[1,18] (with few exceptions[2,12]). In contrast to smooth muscle actin, h-caldesmon is highly specific for smooth muscle differentiation and its negativity argues against a well-developed smooth muscle phenotype in IRMT.[1] The following markers, which are useful in the differential diagnosis, have been systematically tested and shown to be

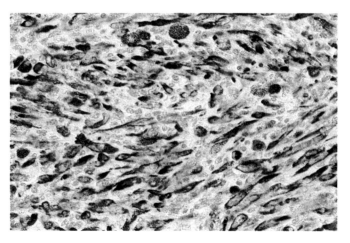

Fig. 6. Desmin is usually diffusely positive in IRMT. Some desmin-positive cells show a histiocyte-like foamy cytoplasm, which is a useful diagnostic clue.

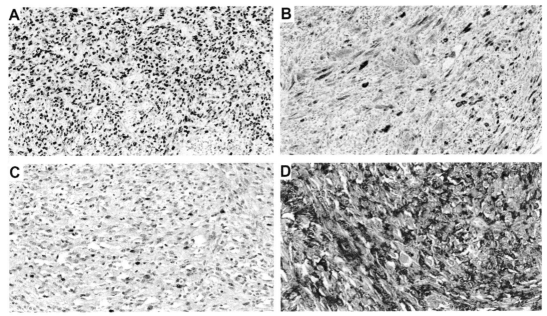

Fig. 7. Although desmin staining tends to be diffuse, the expression of MyoD1, PAX7, and myogenin is usually more limited. Of the latter three, PAX7 tends to show the most extensive expression (*A*), whereas MyoD1 (*B*) and especially myogenin (*C*) often show very focal expression. Besides the aggregates of xanthoma cells, CD163 (*D*) also stains the remarkably high number of spindled histiocytes diffusely admixed among the CD163-negative neoplastic cells. (Photomicrographs courtesy of Andrew L Folpe, M.D., Rochester, Minnesota.).

consistently negative for expression: ALK-1, ROS-1, CD21, CD23, CD34, S100, SOX10, and keratin AE1/3. MDM2 was partially positive by immunohistochemistry in one of seven tested cases, but *MDM2* fluorescence in situ hybridization was negative for gene amplification.[10]

The immunophenotype of the first pattern of progression into RMS showing monomorphic rhabdomyoblastic cell overgrowth is identical to that of conventional IRMT. As noted, to identify the second pattern of progression consisting of high-grade spindled to epithelioid cells as rhabdomyosarcomatous in nature, skeletal muscle markers are necessary; however, expression of desmin, myogenin, and/or MyoD1 may be limited in extent.[2]

MOLECULAR GENETIC FEATURES

As previously discussed, most cases show a near haploid genome with a nonrandom retention of both parental copies of chromosomes 5 and 22 (**Table 3**). A subset of IRMT also retains chromosomes 18 and 20–21, whereas all other autosomes

Table 3 Ancillary studies key features	
Immunohistochemistry-positive	Desmin (usually diffusely positive) PAX7, MyoD1, myogenin (variable, some may be negative) CD163 (diffusely positive in histiocytes) Smooth muscle actin (variable)
Immunohistochemistry-negative	ALK-1, ROS-1, CD21, CD23, CD34, S100, SOX10 and AE1/3, MDM2 (in most cases)
Changes in the chromosomal number	A near haploid genome with a nonrandom retention of both parental copies of chromosomes 5 and 22 A subset of IRMT retains chromosomes 18 and 20–21, whereas all other autosomes usually feature a loss of heterozygosity Some cases also revealed a hyperdiploid karyotype as a consequence of whole genome doubling A subset of cases may lack all these changes
Other recurrent molecular aberrations	Frequent *NF1* gene mutations

feature a loss of heterozygosity (**Fig. 8**). Some studied cases also revealed a hyperdiploid karyotype that is a consequence of whole genome doubling. Nevertheless, even these cases invariably harbored four copies and retained heterozygosity for chromosomes 5 and 22 (and 18, 20–21 in some cases), whereas all remaining autosomes, although being present in two copies, showed loss of heterozygosity.[1,4,6,8,18] Whole genome doubling in near-haploid tumors is thought to represent a rescue event, reducing the deleterious impact of inactivating mutations in crucial genes.[20] However, the distinction of pseudohyperdiploidy from near-haploidy is challenging using current molecular methods.[2] The study of Lee and colleagues[18] used a set of carefully selected fluorescence in situ hybridization probes for genes located on various chromosomes of interest to assess the chromosomal number in IRMT. In this way, they successfully validated their findings previously obtained by Oncoscan (a genome-wide copy number analysis assay). This approach might represent an attractive surrogate method for many pathology laboratories lacking more advanced genetic testing assays to detect chromosomal copy number changes, and to differentiate pseudohyperdiploidy from near-haploidy of tumors.[2]

However, the previously described near-haploid genomic pattern has not been identified in all cases with features consistent with IRMT. A study analyzing four IRMT and reviewing all previously published cases reported that 5 of 22 analyzed IRMT lacked the near-haploid pattern.[18] Whether

cases lacking these genetic changes represent just a genetic variant of IRMT or a fundamentally different entity remains to be defined.[21] However, because cases that were otherwise indistinguishable from the near-haploid IRMT have not followed a more aggressive clinical course in the reported literature[1] and in our unpublished experience, it currently does not seem reasonable to classify them separately.

NF1 gene mutation represents another frequent molecular aberration in IRMT[1,8,10,12,18] and in some of these patients, neurofibromatosis type 1 was clinically confirmed.[1,18] In addition, individual cases of conventional IRMT harbored *ERBB4*, *TP53*, *KRAS*, and *SMARCA4* mutations.[10,12] No recurrent fusion transcripts have been identified.[8–10] As discussed, gene expression profiling revealed highly expressed genes that are known to be crucial for skeletal muscle development, such as *MYOD1*, *MYOG*, *PAX7*, *MYF5*, and *MYF6*, whereas apart from *ACTA2*, genes responsible for smooth muscle differentiation did not show significantly increased expression.[8]

Because of a limited number of published cases, the molecular changes that lead to progression of IRMT into RMS are not entirely clear. As reported by Dehner and colleagues,[2] IRMT exhibiting the first pattern of progression (ie, containing an increased number of monomorphic rhabdomyoblastic cells) showed evidence supporting presumptive pseudohyperdiploidy, with four copies and retained heterozygosity of chromosomes 5 and 20. In contrast, one of the

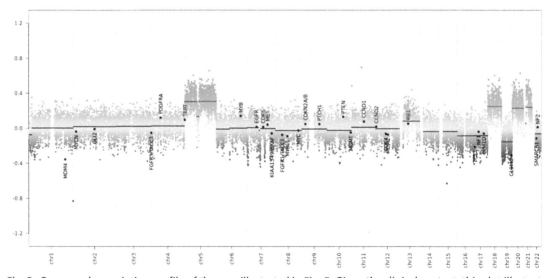

Fig. 8. Copy number variation profile of the case illustrated in **Fig. 5**. Given the clinical context, this plot illustrates a near haploid or pseudohyperdiploid genome (indistinguishable using this method) with retention of both parental copies of chromosomes 5, 18, 20, and 21. Although most cases of IRMT also show loss of chromosome 22, both copies are retained in this case.

analyzed cases allowed for macrodissection and separate analysis of copy number changes in the conventional IRMT areas and in foci with tumor progression. Although both components showed widespread loss of heterozygosity with retained chromosomes 5, 18, and 20–22, only the area with tumor progression revealed evidence of whole genome doubling. This is of interest because, as suggested previously, the whole genome duplication in near-haploid cells might be a predisposing event to subsequent malignant transformation and such molecular events are increasingly recognized as a recurrent pattern in several different malignant neoplasms.[2,20]

In addition to whole genome doubling, areas of rhabdomyosarcomatous progression were also characterized by the presence of additional genomic alterations including a variety of gains and losses. Most importantly, losses involving chromosomes 9p21.3 and/or 9p24.3 were seen in five of six cases, suggesting an important role of these chromosomal regions in the pathogenesis of rhabdomyosarcomatous IRMT.[2] The deletion of genes located on chromosome 9p, including the well-known tumor suppressor genes CDKN2A (p16) and CDKN2B (p15), have been implicated

in a wide variety of human malignancies.[2,22] Additional genetic alterations in the study by Dehner and colleagues[2] included NF1 gene mutations in three of three tested cases. Lastly, besides NF1 and TP53 mutations, one case of rhabdomyosarcomatous IRMT reported by Sukhanova and colleagues[12] also harbored a germline MSH6 gene variant consistent with hereditary nonpolyposis colorectal cancer syndrome (Lynch syndrome).

DIFFERENTIAL DIAGNOSIS

From a morphologic perspective, the differential diagnosis of conventional IRMT may include several entities with overlapping features, such as superficial CD34-positive fibroblastic tumor, inflammatory myofibroblastic tumor, or follicular dendritic cell sarcoma to name a few (Table 4). However, all of these neoplasms are easily distinguished from IRMT based on their negativity for skeletal muscle markers, or by using other appropriate immunostains, such as CD34, follicular dendritic cell markers, or ALK.[10] Therefore, the differential primarily includes morphologically atypical neoplasms with spindled to pleomorphic morphology and skeletal muscle differentiation,

Table 4 Differential diagnosis	
Most important differential diagnostic entities	Spindle cell and pleomorphic rhabdomyosarcoma Other malignant tumors with skeletal muscle immunophenotype (ie, dedifferentiated liposarcoma and melanoma with heterologous skeletal muscle differentiation, other rhabdomyosarcoma subtypes)
Some other potential differential diagnostic entities (based on morphology)	Superficial CD34-positive fibroblastic tumor Inflammatory myofibroblastic tumor Follicular dendritic cell sarcoma
Key differentiating features favoring IRMT	Absence of general features of malignancy: widely infiltrative growth, higher mitotic (>3–4 mitoses/10 high-powered field) and proliferative rate (>10%), large areas of necrosis Presence of a pleomorphic mixture of neoplastic cells Significant and diffuse lymphohistiocytic infiltrate Immunohistochemical expression of skeletal muscle markers and negativity with markers suggestive of other specific diagnosis (ie, ALK) A near haploid genome with a nonrandom retention of both parental copies of chromosomes 5 and 22 with or without subsequent whole genome doubling
Differential diagnosis of rhabdomyosarcoma arising in IRMT	Conventional IRMT areas at the periphery If absent, molecular testing necessary to exclude other rhabdomyosarcoma subtypes

such as dedifferentiated liposarcoma and mela-noma with skeletal muscle differentiation, and spindle cell or pleomorphic RMS.

In general, wide infiltrative growth, higher mitotic (>3–4 mitoses/10 high-power field) and proliferative rate (Ki67 >10%), large areas of ne-crosis, cellular monomorphism (ie, presence of only monotonous spindled cells), and a lack of significant and diffuse lymphohistiocytic infil-trate are all features arguing against the diag-nosis of conventional IRMT in all situations. Rhabdomyoblastic differentiation and corre-sponding expression of desmin and skeletal muscle markers is a rare, but well-recognized feature of dedifferentiated liposarcoma and mel-anoma.[23–25] Besides the previously mentioned general features of high-grade malignancy, both are differentiated in many cases based on clinical history, the presence of better differenti-ated areas, or by using appropriate immunohis-tochemical markers. In most challenging cases, molecular analysis focused on MDM2 copy number status or melanoma-associated genetic changes can be exploited.[25,26] Although the ex-tremity location, pleomorphic mixture of tumor cells, and skeletal muscle immunophenotype may suggest the diagnosis of pleomorphic RMS, these tumors invariably show high-grade malignant features. Lastly, adult spindle cell RMS also enters the differential diagnosis. How-ever, this group currently encompasses several molecular subgroups with slightly different morphology. Although the most common adult spindle cell RMS with MYOD1 mutations has a more monomorphic morphology than IRMT, the affected anatomic locations, age of the pa-tients, and immunophenotype are similar.[27,28] Morphologically, they usually show high-grade spindle cell morphology often with sclerosing areas. It may partially mimic IRMT because of the fascicular arrangement of spindled tumor cells, with a rare admixture of rhabdomyoblasts. However, they usually show signs of a much higher mitotic and proliferative rate and infiltra-tive growth.[29] They also lack the prominent and diffusely present lymphohistiocytic compo-nent, foamy cell aggregates, and the rhabdo-myoblasts of spindle cell RMS, although rarely present, show cross-striations. Although immu-nohistochemistry is largely unhelpful in this dif-ferential diagnosis, MYOD1 mutational analysis may be used for the distinction in morphologi-cally challenging cases. The recently described spindle cell and epithelioid RMS with EWSR1::TFCP2 or FUS::TFCP2 fusion typically arise in craniofacial bones but may also affect soft tissue sites. Besides skeletal muscle immunophenotype, these tumors are often diffusely positive with cytokeratins and often overexpress ALK.[30] Other fusion-positive adult RMS subgroups, including cases with NCOA2, NCOA3, and VGLL3 fusions, and those RMS lacking any identifiable molecular aberrations, typically show a highly monomorphic spindle cell proliferation usually with infiltrative growth pattern, variable but often high mitotic activity, and absence of prominent inflammatory infil-trate.[31–33] Aside from morphology, the poten-tially challenging differential diagnosis with regard to spindle cell RMS versus IRMT would benefit from identification of recurrent molecular abnormalities seen in spindle cell RMS or, alter-natively, the near-haploid genome of IRMT.

The differential diagnostic approach to RMS arising in IRMT depends on the presence or absence of conventional IRMT areas. If the latter component is absent, a confident diagnosis, and distinction particularly from pleomorphic and some spindle cell RMS subtypes, is impossible without identifying the characteristic genomic fea-tures of IRMT.[2]

SUMMARY AND FUTURE DIRECTIONS

IRMT has been an excellent example of how surgi-cal pathologists working in conjunction with tumor biologists can greatly improve tumor classification to the benefit of patients. Because of this prog-ress, it is now known that tumors formerly routinely diagnosed as high-grade malignancies are in fact mostly indolent tumors adequately treated by sur-gery. Pathologists are also starting to learn how to identify the significant minority of cases with the potential for aggressive behavior. However, there is still undoubtedly much to learn about this intriguing neoplasm. There are several areas of in-terest for future research, such as defining the pre-cise morphologic or molecular criteria for identifying cases progressing or at risk for pro-gression to RMS, assessing the relationship be-tween cases with and without the near-haploid genome, more precisely characterizing the associ-ation of IRMT with tumor syndromes, and identi-fying the optimal therapy for clinically aggressive cases. Future studies with additional cases of con-ventional and particularly rhabdomyosarcomatous IRMT are needed to answer these remaining questions.

DISCLOSURE

The author has nothing to disclose.

CLINICS CARE POINTS

- Often focal expression of MyoD1 and especially myogenin in IRMT.
- Lack of near-haploid genome in a minor subset of IRMT despite typical morphological features.
- A subset of IRMT may progress to RMS, warranting a thorough sampling and a careful morphological assessment of all sections.

FUNDING

This study was supported by the Cooperatio program, research area SURG.

ACKNOWLEDGMENT

The author thanks A.L. Folpe, MD, Rochester, Minnesota, who kindly provided photomicrographs for **Fig. 4**.

REFERENCES

1. Cloutier JM, Charville GW, Mertens F, et al. Inflammatory Leiomyosarcoma" and "Histiocyte-rich Rhabdomyoblastic Tumor": a clinicopathological, immunohistochemical and genetic study of 13 cases, with a proposal for reclassification as "Inflammatory Rhabdomyoblastic Tumor. Mod Pathol 2021; 34:758–69.

2. Dehner CA, Geiersbach K, Rowsey R, et al. Rhabdomyosarcoma Arising in Inflammatory Rhabdomyoblastic Tumor: A Genetically Distinctive Subtype of Rhabdomyosarcoma. Mod Pathol 2023;36:100131.

3. Merchant W, Calonje E, Fletcher CD. Inflammatory leiomyosarcoma: a morphological subgroup within the heterogeneous family of so-called inflammatory malignant fibrous histiocytoma. Histopathology 1995;27:525–32.

4. Dal Cin P, Sciot R, Fletcher CD, et al. Inflammatory leiomyosarcoma may be characterized by specific near-haploid chromosome changes. J Pathol 1998; 185:112–5.

5. Chang A, Schuetze SM, Conrad EU 3rd, et al. So-called "inflammatory leiomyosarcoma": a series of 3 cases providing additional insights into a rare entity. Int J Surg Pathol 2005;13:185–95.

6. Nord KH, Paulsson K, Veerla S, et al. Retained heterodisomy is associated with high gene expression in hyperhaploid inflammatory leiomyosarcoma. Neoplasia 2012;14:807–12.

7. de Saint Aubain Somerhausen N, Gengler C, Reginster M, et al. [Inflammatory leiomyosarcoma: a case report]. Ann Pathol 2003;23:336–9.

8. Arbajian E, Koster J, Vult von Steyern F, et al. Inflammatory leiomyosarcoma is a distinct tumor characterized by near-haploidization, few somatic mutations, and a primitive myogenic gene expression signature. Mod Pathol 2018;31:93–100.

9. Martinez AP, Fritchie KJ, Weiss SW, et al. Histiocyte-rich rhabdomyoblastic tumor: rhabdomyosarcoma, rhabdomyoma, or rhabdomyoblastic tumor of uncertain malignant potential? A histologically distinctive rhabdomyoblastic tumor in search of a place in the classification of skeletal muscle neoplasms. Mod Pathol 2019;32:446–57.

10. Michal M, Rubin BP, Kazakov DV, et al. Inflammatory leiomyosarcoma shows frequent co-expression of smooth and skeletal muscle markers supporting a primitive myogenic phenotype: a report of 9 cases with a proposal for reclassification as low-grade inflammatory myogenic tumor. Virchows Arch 2020; 477:219–30.

11. Geiersbach K, Kleven DT, Blankenship HT, et al. Inflammatory rhabdomyoblastic tumor with progression to high-grade rhabdomyosarcoma. Mod Pathol 2021;34:1035–6.

12. Sukhanova M, Obeidin F, Streich L, et al. Inflammatory leiomyosarcoma/rhabdomyoblastic tumor: A report of two cases with novel genetic findings. Genes Chromosomes Cancer 2022;61:653–61.

13. Bell D, Phan J, DeMonte F, et al. High-grade transformation of low-grade biphenotypic sinonasal sarcoma: Radiological, morphophenotypic variation and confirmatory molecular analysis. Ann Diagn Pathol 2022;57:151889.

14. Hasnie S, Glenn C, Peterson JEG, et al. High-Grade Biphenotypic Sinonasal Sarcoma: A Case Report. J Neurol Surg Rep 2022;83:e105–9.

15. Meyer A, Klubickova N, Mosaieby E, et al. Biphenotypic sinonasal sarcoma with PAX3::MAML3 fusion transforming into high-grade rhabdomyosarcoma: report of an emerging rare phenomenon. Virchows Arch 2023;482:777–82.

16. Kao YC, Kuo CT, Kuo PY, et al. Pulmonary "Inflammatory Leiomyosarcomas" Are Indolent Tumors With Diploid Genomes and No Convincing Rhabdomyoblastic Differentiation. Am J Surg Pathol 2022; 46:424–33.

17. Rekhi B, Bal M, Dharavath B, et al. A Rare Case of A Low-Grade Inflammatory Leiomyosarcoma/Histiocyte-Rich Rhabdomyoblastic Tumor in the Neck of An Adolescent Male. Turk Patoloji Derg 2023;39(2): 154–60.

18. Lee JC, Li WS, Kao YC, et al. Toward a unifying entity that encompasses most, but perhaps not all, inflammatory leiomyosarcomas and histiocyte-rich

rhabdomyoblastic tumors. Mod Pathol 2021;34: 1434–8.

19. Bourgeau M, Martinez AP. Histiocyte-rich rhabdomyoblastic tumor: a report of two cases and a review of the differential diagnoses. Virchows Arch 2021; 478:367–73.

20. Cortes-Ciriano I, Steele CD, Piculell K, et al. Genomic Patterns of Malignant Peripheral Nerve Sheath Tumor (MPNST) Evolution Correlate with Clinical Outcome and Are Detectable in Cell-Free DNA. Cancer Discov 2023;13:654–71.

21. Folpe AL. Response to Lee et al: Toward a unifying entity that encompasses most, but perhaps not all, inflammatory leiomyosarcomas and histiocyte-rich rhabdomyoblastic tumors. Mod Pathol 2021;34: 1439.

22. Goncalves PG, Reis RM, Bidinotto LT. Significance of Chr9p22.1-p21.3 Deletion in Cancer Development: A Pan-cancer In Silico Analysis. Anticancer Res 2022;42:5291–304.

23. Salzano RP Jr, Tomkiewicz Z, Africano WA. Dedifferentiated liposarcoma with features of rhabdomyosarcoma. Conn Med 1991;55:200–2.

24. Tallini G, Erlandson RA, Brennan MF, et al. Divergent myosarcomatous differentiation in retroperitoneal liposarcoma. Am J Surg Pathol 1993;17:546–56.

25. Agaimy A, Stoehr R, Hornung A, et al. Dedifferentiated and Undifferentiated Melanomas: Report of 35 New Cases With Literature Review and Proposal of Diagnostic Criteria. Am J Surg Pathol 2021;45: 240–54.

26. Kasago IS, Chatila WK, Lezcano CM, et al. Undifferentiated and Dedifferentiated Metastatic Melanomas Masquerading as Soft Tissue Sarcomas: Mutational Signature Analysis and Immunotherapy Response. Mod Pathol 2023;36:100165.

27. Kohsaka S, Shukla N, Ameur N, et al. A recurrent neomorphic mutation in MYOD1 defines a clinically aggressive subset of embryonal rhabdomyosarcoma associated with PI3K-AKT pathway mutations. Nat Genet 2014;46:595–600.

28. Alaggio R, Zhang L, Sung YS, et al. A Molecular Study of Pediatric Spindle and Sclerosing Rhabdomyosarcoma: Identification of Novel and Recurrent VGLL2-related Fusions in Infantile Cases. Am J Surg Pathol 2016;40:224–35.

29. Leiner J, Le Loarer F. The current landscape of rhabdomyosarcomas: an update. Virchows Arch 2020; 476:97–108.

30. Le Loarer F, Cleven AHG, Bouvier C, et al. A subset of epithelioid and spindle cell rhabdomyosarcomas is associated with TFCP2 fusions and common ALK upregulation. Mod Pathol 2020;33:404–19.

31. Agaimy A, Dermawan JK, Leong I, et al. Recurrent VGLL3 fusions define a distinctive subset of spindle cell rhabdomyosarcoma with an indolent clinical course and striking predilection for the head and neck. Genes Chromosomes Cancer 2022;61:701–9.

32. Agaram NP, Zhang L, Sung YS, et al. Expanding the Spectrum of Intraosseous Rhabdomyosarcoma: Correlation Between 2 Distinct Gene Fusions and Phenotype. Am J Surg Pathol 2019;43:695–702.

33. Han R, Dermawan JK, Demicco EG, et al. ZFP64::NCOA3 gene fusion defines a novel subset of spindle cell rhabdomyosarcoma. Genes Chromosomes Cancer 2022;61:645–52.

Calcified Chondroid Mesenchymal Neoplasms

Erica Y. Kao, MD[a], Eleanor Y. Chen, MD, PhD[b],*

KEYWORDS

- Chondroblastoma-like soft tissue chondroma • Chondroid tenosynovial giant cell tumor
- Tophaceous pseudogout / tumoral calcium pyrophosphate dihydrate crystal deposition disease
- Calcified chondroid mesenchymal neoplasm

> **Key points**
>
> - Calcified chondroid mesenchymal neoplasms represent a family of chondroid matrix-producing tumors characterized by lobular growth of ovoid to stellate cells within chondroid matrix with calcifications and harboring an *FN1* gene fusion to a receptor tyrosine kinase.
>
> - Includes entities currently classified as chondroid TGCT, chondroblastoma-like soft tissue chondroma, and cellular examples of tophaceous pseudogout.
>
> - These tumors are benign with potential for recurrence.

ABSTRACT

Calcified chondroid mesenchymal neoplasms (CCMN) represent a morphologic spectrum of related tumors. Historically, chondroid matrix or chondroblastoma-like features have been described in soft tissue chondroma, tenosynovial giant cell tumors (especially of the temporomandibular joint (TMJ) region), and in a subset of tophaceous pseudogout. Recently, these tumors have been found to share FN1-receptor tyrosine kinase (RTK) fusions. This review discusses the clinical, morphologic, immunohistochemical, and molecular genetic features of CCMN. The distinction from morphologic mimics is also discussed.

OVERVIEW

Recently, it has been recognized that a subset of soft tissue neoplasms with calcifying chondroid matrix production harbor specific FN1-Receptor Tyrosine Kinase (RTK) fusions.[1,2] The described tumors with FN1::RTK fusion show a range of morphologies but have certain features in common; namely, chondroblastoma-like matrix production, a proliferation of ovoid to spindled cells with occasional osteoclast-like giant cells, and a lobular growth pattern. In their 2001 study of 17 cases of the distal upper extremity, Cates and colleagues were the first to describe a chondroblastoma-like variant of soft tissue chondroma where they noted that a subset of chondromas displayed cellular foci composed of polygonal to elongate chondroblastic cells admixed with variable numbers of osteoclast-like multinucleated giant cells and coarse, granular calcifications or even lace-like, chicken wire calcification patterns. Since that time, there have been continued case reports of chondroblastoma-like chondromas of soft tissue in the extremities and head and neck region.[3–5]

Besides soft tissue chondroma, similar calcifying matrix production has been noted in giant cell-rich tumors, especially in the temporomandibular joint (TMJ) region, and termed chondroid tenosynovial giant cell tumors (TGCT) or TGCT with chondroid metaplasia.[6–11] In 2011, Hoch and colleagues observed in their study of 5 cases in the TMJ region that these tumors had a mononuclear cell proliferation, multinucleated giant cells, and chondroid matrix formation to include lace-like intercellular calcification similar to that seen in chondroblastoma, but had an absence of sheets or aggregates of foamy histiocytes.[9] As the cells within the

[a] Department of Pathology, Brooke Army Medical Center, 3551 Roger Brooke Drive, Building 3600, 4th Floor, Room 447-6, San Antonio, TX 78234, USA; [b] Department of Laboratory Medicine and Pathology, University of Washington, 1959 Northeast Pacific Street, Box 357705, HSB Room K072A, Seattle, WA 98195-7705, USA
* Corresponding author.
E-mail address: eleanor2@uw.edu

Surgical Pathology 17 (2024) 77–82
https://doi.org/10.1016/j.path.2023.06.006

chondroid component were considered similar to the larger mononuclear cells in conventional TGCT, these tumors were thought to represent TGCT with chondroid metaplasia. Carlson and colleagues (in 2017) and Wang and colleagues (in 2019) described additional cases of TGCT in the TMJ region with chondroid metaplasia and chondroblastoma-like features to include an epithelioid tumor cell population associated with calcification. In both series of cases, the authors noticed erosion of the adjacent bone.[10,12]

Furthermore, the chondromas and TGCTs mentioned above have been noted to be heavily mineralized with areas resembling crystal deposition disease, while some tumors were noted to be associated with bona fide calcium pyrophosphate deposition (CPPD) crystals.[1,9,13] In the past, others have noticed the association of chondroid matrix-producing tumors with calcium pyrophosphate crystal deposition,[14,15] particularly in the TMJ region, and called it tophaceous pseudogout, although on closer inspection of the histology, these tumors appeared too cellular for true crystal deposition disease. Ishida and colleagues noted calcium pyrophosphate deposition in both the extremity and TMJ region that was mass-forming and called it tophaceous pseudogout. However, a subset of the cases included in their series also demonstrated increased cellularity more than would be expected for a pure crystal deposition disease. The association of CPPD crystals with chondroid matrix calcification certainly complicates matters and blurs the distinction between soft tissue chondroma, chondroid TGCT, and cellular tophaceous pseudogout.

In all the series mentioned thus far, the tumors exhibited lobular architecture, contained cells with ovoid to spindled cytomorphology, had flocculent or grungy calcification resembling chondroblastoma or CPPD deposition, and occurred in the extremity or TMJ region. It was not until the 2019 study by Amary and colleagues when it was noticed that this "subset of soft tissue chondromas characterized by grungy calcification, a feature reminiscent of phosphaturic mesenchymal tumor" harbored *FN1::FGFR1/2* fusions.[1] The range of reported morphologic findings suggests that these tumors encompass a related family of neoplasms with shared molecular findings and a benign clinical behavior. In 2021, to clarify this issue, Liu and colleagues studied 12 of these calcifying chondroid matrix-producing tumors and showed the overwhelming majority of these tumors shared an *FN1* fusion to *FGFR1*, *FGFR2*, *MERTK*, *NTRK1*, and *TEK*, which are all genes encoding receptor tyrosine kinases.[2]

The term "calcified chondroid mesenchymal neoplasm" (CCMN) is a useful umbrella term that captures the morphologic spectrum of these entities. The shared molecular finding of *FN1* fused to a receptor tyrosine kinase and similar benign clinical behavior and overlapping morphologies supports the concept that CCMN is a spectrum of related entities. This article will review the clinical, histopathologic, and molecular features of CCMN with particular attention to their distinction from other chondroid mesenchymal tumors.

CLINICAL FEATURES

Most CCMNs present as soft tissue masses in the distal extremities or TMJ region and occur generally in the adult population with a mean age of 55.7 (range 22–72 years).[2] To date, these tumors have not been described in the pediatric population. Tumors range in size from 0.5 to 4.0 cm (mean 3.1 cm) and occur in both males and females with no apparent gender predilection.[2] Bony erosion has been noted in some cases, particularly in the TMJ region[2,12,15].

GROSS AND MICROSCOPIC FEATURES

Tumors consist of a multinodular growth of ovoid aggregates containing white-tan firm to gritty tissue, depending on the extent of calcification. All of the tumors have the following features in common: multinodular architecture, chondroid to cartilaginous matrix, and an ovoid to stellate cell proliferation (**Figs.** 1A–D and 2A–D). The matrix can show varying types of calcification from coarse or grungy to lace-like and pericellular (**Fig.** 1B, E). In some cases, the calcifications are basophilic and crystalline with a component of calcium pyrophosphate crystal deposition (CPPD) (**Fig.** 1E, F). The tumor cells embedded within the matrix are ovoid to spindled, while cells in fibrous septa tend to be smaller and spindled with fibroblastic features. Tumors often have increased cellularity toward the periphery of the nodules. Osteoclast-like giant cells and histiocytoid or ovoid cells resembling tenosynovial giant cell tumor cells are present in some cases (see **Fig.** 2D).

IMMUNOHISTOCHEMISTRY

The immunophenotype is not specific and generally not helpful in the diagnosis, which is based on morphology and molecular studies, if the morphologic features are not characteristic. The cells may be variably or focally positive for S100 protein in chondroid areas as has been previously described in chondroid matrix-producing tumors. Tumors that fall under chondroid tenosynovial giant cell tumor may express Clusterin in larger mononuclear cells and Desmin in dendritic-like cells.

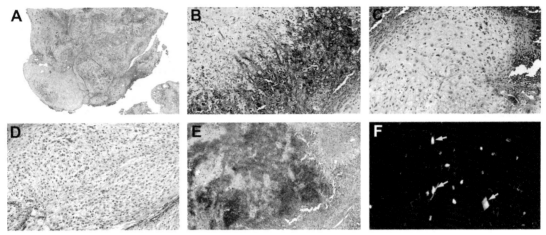

Fig. 1. Histologic features of CCMNs with *FN1::FGFR2* fusion. (*A*) Characteristic lobular architecture at low power. (*B*) Grungy to lacy (chondroblastoma-like) calcifications. (*C, D*) Polygonal, ovoid to spindled cells within the chondroid matrix frequently associated with osteoclast-like giant cells. (*E*) Case with extensive basophilic grungy calcification at low power with CPPD crystalline deposits. (*F*) Refractile rhomboid crystals (some indicated by *arrows*) of the same case in E when viewed using polarized light.

MOLECULAR FEATURES

At the molecular genetic level, the majority of CCMN show *FN1::FGFR2* fusions. Other *FN1* fusion partners that have been described include *FGFR1, MERTK, TEK,* and *NTRK1,*[1,2] which are all genes that encode for receptor tyrosine kinases. *FN1* encodes fibronectin-1, a glycoprotein usually present in dimeric form, which plays a major role in the extracellular matrix (ECM) and in signal

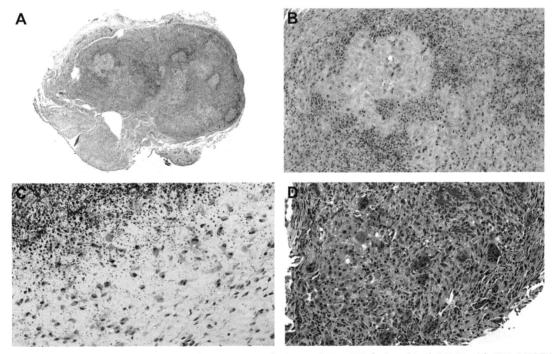

Fig. 2. Histologic features of CCMNs with *FN1::MERTK* fusion and *FN1::TEK* fusion. (*A, B*) CCMN with *FN1::MERTK* fusion, showing vaguely lobular architecture with circumscribed tumor border (*A*). Cells within the variably chondroid matrix and collagenous stroma are polygonal to oval with eosinophilic cytoplasm and eccentrically placed nuclei (*B*). (*C, D*) CCMN with *FN1::TEK* fusion with focal area of epithelioid to stellate cells in a chondroid matrix with calcification (*C*). Other areas show ovoid cells with eccentric nuclei admixed with osteoclast-like giant cells, resembling tenosynovial giant cell tumor (*D*).

transduction.[16] Each monomer of the molecule contains different numbers of repeating type 1, 2, and 3 binding domains, which allows for interaction with many other ECM proteins as well as small molecules, growth factors, glycosaminoglycans, cell surface receptors, and other fibronectin molecules. Receptor tyrosine kinases are a subclass of tyrosine kinases involved in mediating cell-to-cell communication. The dysregulation of receptor tyrosine kinases is a known pathway of tumorigenesis, and one of the principal mechanisms for abnormal activation is chromosomal rearrangement.[17]

The fusions in CCMN result in the in-frame fusion of the N-terminal region of FN1 containing the signal peptide and the FN1 type 1 to 3 domains to the intact transmembrane and TK domains of the RTK (example schematics in **Fig. 3**), which is hypothesized to promote the dimerization of the fused receptor through the fibronectin (FN) domain and lead to enhanced signal activation.

DIFFERENTIAL DIAGNOSIS

Other chondroid matrix-forming neoplasms harboring *FN1* rearrangements with which CCMN may be confused include phosphaturic mesenchymal tumor (PMT), synovial chondromatosis (SCM), and calcifying aponeurotic fibroma (CAF).

Phosphaturic mesenchymal tumors have a range of morphologic features, but many are characterized by a grungy pattern of calcification in a chondroosseous matrix and often contain osteoclast-like giant cells. They tend to have a mixture of bland spindled to stellate cells and vascular stroma.[18] PMTs typically present with metabolic disturbances involving hypophosphatemia, and usually have symptoms of tumor-induced osteomalacia (TIO)

such as bone pain and multiple fractures. They are characterized by *FN1::FGFR1* gene fusions, or less commonly, *FN1::FGF1*,[19,20] and have high *FGF23* mRNA expression. In contrast to CCMN, PMT retains the Ig domains in FGFR1 that enable the interactions of the fusion protein with FGF23 [2]. *FGF23* expression by chromogenic in situ hybridization (CISH) or RT-PCR can be useful as both CCMN and PMTs share *FN1::FGFR1* gene fusions, especially in distinguishing CCMN from PMT without clinically apparent TIO. CCMNs do not have high levels of *FGF23* mRNA expression.

Synovial chondromatosis is characterized by the formation of multiple nodules of mature, hyaline cartilage with clustered groups of chondrocytes sitting in well-formed lacunae. It is closely associated with the articular joints and synovium, while soft tissue chondromas by definition are not related to the synovial lining. This tumor harbors an *FN1::ACVR2A* rearrangement, and may undergo malignant transformation.[1]

Another type of tumor with recurrent *FN1* gene rearrangements is calcifying aponeurotic fibroma (CAF). It typically affects the palms and soles of children and young adults, has a more infiltrative growth pattern, and the calcification pattern is different as it is linear and punctate as opposed to a broader area of distribution. This tumor harbors recurrent *FN1::EGF* fusions, and is thought to be related to a subset of lipofibromatosis due to the shared fusion.[21,22]

Additionally, acral fibrochondromyxoid tumor (AFCMT), a recently described matrix-producing tumor with a predilection for the acral region may also be on the differential. These tumors show significant overlap in histomorphologic features with CCMN, although this type of tumor

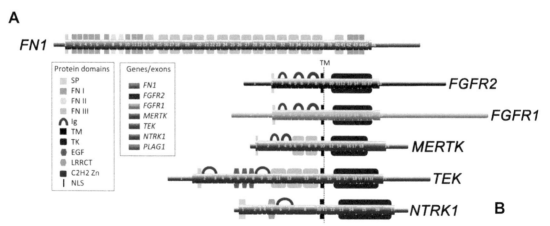

Fig. 3. Schematic of chimeric transcripts and proteins resulting from gene fusions. (*A*). RNA transcripts with exon structures and related protein domains in the genes involved in the fusions. (*B*). Chimeric transcripts and proteins detected in CCMNs, showing the retained exons and functional domains of the fusion genes of *FN1, FGFR2, FGFR1, MERTK, TEK* and *NTRK1*.

tends to have a distinct stroma that is fibrous or chondromyxoid and harbors a *THBS1::ADGRF5* gene fusion.[23]

DIAGNOSIS

- Hinges on key histologic features: presence of ovoid to spindled cells within chondroid to grungy matrix displaying lobular growth with occasional osteoclast-like giant cells.
- Immunohistochemistry generally not useful
- Molecular testing (targeted RNA sequencing, eg, targeted fusion gene panel) for FN1::RTK fusions to help distinguish from histologic mimics.

PROGNOSIS

Recurrences do occur after complete or incomplete surgical excision, but seem to be infrequent. The recurrence rates appear to be similar across the spectrum of tumors although it is not clear if all of these cases represent complete or incomplete surgical excisions and there is limited follow-up data available. Cates and colleagues reported a recurrence rate of 1 out of 6 (17%) for patients with marginal excisions of chondromas with available follow-up data.[13] Hoch and colleagues reported 1 out of 5 patients with recurrent disease for chondroid TGCT.[9] Ishida and colleagues reported 1 out of 5 patients with recurrences on 2 occasions for tophaceous pseudogout.[24] None of the cases reported evidence of metastatic disease.

SUMMARY

CCMN is a clinicopathologically and genetically distinct family of tumors with a predilection for the distal extremities and TMJ region. Awareness of the morphologic spectrum of this entity and ancillary testing for FN1::RTK fusions in select cases, allows for the distinction from other matrix-producing tumors of soft tissue. These neoplasms are benign, generally amenable to surgical excision, and have no documented metastasis although they may recur.

CLINICS CARE POINTS

- Most cases present as small soft tissue masses in the distal extremity or TMJ region in adult patients.

- There have been no reports of malignant behavior. Conservative surgical management is adequate.

DISCLOSURE

The authors have nothing to disclose.

REFERENCES

1. Amary F, Perez-Casanova L, Ye H, et al. Synovial chondromatosis and soft tissue chondroma: extra-osseous cartilaginous tumor defined by FN1 gene rearrangement. Mod Pathol 2019;32(12):1762–71.
2. Liu YJ, Wang W, Yeh J, et al. Calcified chondroid mesenchymal neoplasms with FN1-receptor tyrosine kinase gene fusions including FGFR2, FGFR1, MERTK, NTRK1, and TEK: a molecular and clinico-pathologic analysis. Mod Pathol 2021;34(7):1373–83.
3. Raparia K, Lin JW, Donovan D, et al. Chondroblastoma-like chondroma of soft tissue: report of the first case in the base of skull. Ann Diagn Pathol 2013; 17(3):298–301.
4. AlYami AH. Chondroblastoma-Like Soft-Tissue Chondroma of the Hand: A Case Report. Cureus 2021;13(11):e19467.
5. Kuprys TK, Bindra R, Borys D, et al. Chondroblastoma-like chondroma of the hand: case report. J Hand Surg Am 2014;39(5):933–6.
6. Oda Y, Izumi T, Harimaya K, et al. Pigmented villonodular synovitis with chondroid metaplasia, resembling chondroblastoma of the bone: a report of three cases. Mod Pathol 2007;20(5):545–51.
7. Anbinder AL, Geraldo BMC, Guimarães R, et al. Chondroid Tenosynovial Giant Cell Tumor of the Temporomandibular Joint: A Rare Case Report. Braz Dent J 2017;28(5):647–52.
8. Pina S, Fernandez M, Maya S, et al. Recurrent temporal bone tenosynovial giant cell tumor with chondroid metaplasia: the use of imaging to assess recurrence. NeuroRadiol J 2014;27(1):97–101.
9. Hoch BL, Garcia RA, Smalberger GJ. Chondroid tenosynovial giant cell tumor: a clinicopathological and immunohistochemical analysis of 5 new cases. Int J Surg Pathol 2011;19(2):180–7.
10. Carlson ML, Osetinsky LM, Alon EE, et al. Tenosynovial giant cell tumors of the temporomandibular joint and lateral skull base: Review of 11 cases. Laryngoscope 2017;127(10):2340–6.
11. Fisher M, Biddinger P, Folpe AL, et al. Chondroid tenosynovial giant cell tumor of the temporal bone. Otol Neurotol 2013;34(6):e49–50.
12. Wang JG, Liu J, He B, et al. Diffuse Tenosynovial Giant Cell Tumor Around the Temporomandibular Joint: An Entity With Special Radiologic and Pathologic Features. J Oral Maxillofac Surg 2019;77(5):1022, e1-e39.
13. Cates JM, Rosenberg AE, O'Connell JX, et al. Chondroblastoma-like chondroma of soft tissue: an underrecognized variant and its differential diagnosis. Am J Surg Pathol 2001;25(5):661–6.

14. Kurihara K, Mizuseki K, Saiki T, et al. Tophaceous pseudogout of the temporomandibular joint: report of a case. Pathol Int 1997;47(8):578–80.

15. Houghton D, Munir N, Triantafyllou A, et al. Tophaceous pseudogout of the temporomandibular joint with erosion into the middle cranial fossa. Int J Oral Maxillofac Surg 2020. https://doi.org/10.1016/j.ijom.2020.03.011.

16. Dalton CJ, Lemmon CA. Fibronectin: Molecular Structure, Fibrillar Structure and Mechanochemical Signaling. Cells 2021;10(9):2443.

17. Du Z, Lovly CM. Mechanisms of receptor tyrosine kinase activation in cancer. Mol Cancer 2018;17(1):58.

18. Folpe AL, Fanburg-Smith JC, Billings SD, et al. Most osteomalacia-associated mesenchymal tumors are a single histopathologic entity: an analysis of 32 cases and a comprehensive review of the literature. Am J Surg Pathol 2004;28(1):1–30.

19. Lee JC, Jeng YM, Su SY, et al. Identification of a novel FN1-FGFR1 genetic fusion as a frequent event in phosphaturic mesenchymal tumour. J Pathol 2015;235(4):539–45.

20. Bahrami A, Weiss SW, Montgomery E, et al. RT-PCR analysis for FGF23 using paraffin sections in the diagnosis of phosphaturic mesenchymal tumors with and without known tumor induced osteomalacia. Am J Surg Pathol 2009;33(9):1348–54.

21. Puls F, Hofvander J, Magnusson L, et al. FN1-EGF gene fusions are recurrent in calcifying aponeurotic fibroma. J Pathol 2016;238(4):502–7.

22. Al-Ibraheemi A, Folpe AL, Perez-Atayde AR, et al. Aberrant receptor tyrosine kinase signaling in lipofibromatosis: a clinicopathological and molecular genetic study of 20 cases. Mod Pathol 2019;32(3):423–34.

23. Bouvier C, Le Loarer F, Macagno N, et al. Recurrent novel THBS1-ADGRF5 gene fusion in a new tumor subtype "Acral FibroChondroMyxoid Tumors.". Mod Pathol 2020;33(7):1360–8.

24. Ishida T, Dorfman HD, Bullough PG. Tophaceous pseudogout (tumoral calcium pyrophosphate dihydrate crystal deposition disease). Hum Pathol 1995;26(6):587–93.

Myxoinflammatory Fibroblastic Sarcoma

Hao Wu, MD, PhD, William B. Laskin, MD*

KEYWORDS

- Myxoinflammatory fibroblastic sarcoma • Virocyte-like cells • Reed-Sternberg-like cells
- Pseudolipoblasts • Emperipolesis

Key points

- Conventional MIFS is a low-grade fibroblastic sarcoma with recurrent but minimal metastatic potential that predilects to superficial soft tissues of the distal extremity.
- MIFS consists of plump spindled and epithelioid cells, inflammatory infiltrates, and mucin deposits in a fibrosclerotic stroma.
- Two characteristic ("hallmark") cells are large epithelioid cells harboring bizarre nuclei and virocyte-like macronucleoli and pleomorphic pseudolipoblasts.
- Immunohistochemistry and molecular profiling currently play a limited role in diagnosis.
- Wide local excision is the treatment of choice.

ABSTRACT

MIFS is a low-grade fibroblastic sarcoma that predilects to superficial distal extremity soft tissue. It is composed of plump spindled and epithelioid cells, inflammatory infiltrates, and mucin deposits in a fibrosclerotic stroma. Large epithelioid cells harboring bizarre nuclei and virocyte-like macronucleoli and pleomorphic pseudolipoblasts are characteristic. While conventional MIFS has locally recurrent potential but minimal metastatic risk, tumors with high-grade histologic features have a greater risk for recurrence and metastasis. Wide local excision is the recommended treatment.

OVERVIEW

Myxoinflammatory fibroblastic sarcoma (MIFS) is a low-grade fibroblastic sarcoma with a predilection for the superficial distal extremity soft tissue that exhibits recurrent potential and minimal risk for metastatic spread. The clinicopathologic features of the lesion were first delineated in 1998 by three separate groups[1–3] who emphasized its acral location and striking histologic attributes. As the entity is now known to also occur in non-acral sites, the World Health Organization adopted the term "myxoinflammatory fibroblastic sarcoma."

Clinically, MIFS presents in adults with a peak incidence in the 4th through 6th decades of life and shows no sex predilection.[4–6] Rare pediatric cases have been reported.[2,7–9] The tumor arises predominantly in the dorsal superficial soft tissue of the distal extremities, most commonly the hands and fingers.[4–6] Non-acral extremity sites, limb girdles, trunk, and head/face account for over 40% of cases.[4–6] The lesions are typically slow-growing and asymptomatic, with less than 20% of patients complaining of tumor-related symptoms.[1,5,6] Symptom duration ranges from weeks to "years"[1,5] with most patients presenting within 1 year.[5] MRI imaging is non-specific and demonstrates a poorly circumscribed, multinodular mass which is T1 hypo/isointense, T2 intermediate/hyperintense[10,11] and often shows diffuse postcontrast enhancement on T1.[10] High-grade variants of MIFS have been noted to invade bone radiologically.[12]

Department of Pathology, Yale University School of Medicine, New Haven, CT 06520, USA
* Corresponding author.
E-mail address: william.laskin@yale.edu

Surgical Pathology 17 (2024) 83–96
https://doi.org/10.1016/j.path.2023.07.003
1875-9181/24/

GROSS FEATURES

The tumors average 3-4 cm (range: 0.5 to 30 cm) in greatest dimension.[4–6,13] Proximal extremity and truncal tumors tend to be larger than those of the distal extremity. Most tumors center in the subcutaneous fat, extend into the dermis, and track along deep fascia and tendon sheaths (**Fig. 1**). The tumor is typically lobulated or nodular and poorly circumscribed with a firm to rubbery consistency. The cut surfaces are solid to myxoid, light tan-gray to yellow-pink with rare cysts, foci of hemorrhage, or necrosis.[4–6]

MICROSCOPIC FEATURES

- Microscopically, the tumor is composed of four intermingled elements in varying proportions: epithelioid and spindled tumor cells, mucin, inflammatory cells, and fibrosclerotic stroma **Fig. 2**A).[1–3,5] At low-power magnification, most cases exhibit an inflamed and variably cellular fibrosclerotic stroma interrupted by small mucin-rich pools (**Fig. 2B**). Large mucin lakes are less common.[5] Tenosynovium involvement often manifests as bulbous, myxoedematous fronds with lesional elements (**Fig. 2C**).[1,5]
- The main neoplastic element consists of epithelioid and spindle cells. The epithelioid cells have vesicular nuclei with conspicuous nucleoli, and fibrillary or ground-glass cytoplasm with distinct cell borders (**Fig. 3A**). Plump, mildly atypical, spindled cells with fibrillary cytoplasm often arranged in short fascicles are a minor cellular component (**Fig. 3B**). Both cell types can have binucleation or multiple fused nuclei.

- Two distinct cell types found in varying numbers constitute "hallmark" cells of MIFS. The most characteristic is the "Reed-Sternberg (RS)-like cell" (**Fig. 4A**). This is a large epithelioid cell with abundant deeply eosinophilic cytoplasm and an enlarged, irregularly contoured nucleus with vesicular chromatin and a viral inclusion-like eosinophilic macronucleolus (resembling true RS cells). RS-like cells may occasionally have smudgy heterochromatin resembling a mummified RS cell (**Fig. 4B**). The other "hallmark" cell, the "pseudolipoblast" (**Fig. 4C**), has a pleomorphic nucleus and abundant cytoplasm distended by mucin-filled vacuoles. Pseudolipoblasts are mostly found within mucinous areas.[1–3,5,6,13]
- Epithelioid cells exhibiting emperipolesis with a variable number of intracytoplasmic inflammatory cells, mostly polymorphonuclear leukocytes,[13] are common, but usually in sparse numbers (**Fig. 4D**).
- Pools and larger lakes of mucin are visible at low-power magnification and often harbor loosely organized, cords and trabeculae of lesional cells slightly separated by intercellular mucin (**Fig. 5**). In solid cellular foci, mucin is observed gently separating lesional cells and forming small deposits (see **Fig. 3A**).
- The inflammatory component consists primarily of lymphocytes and plasma cells forming aggregates and lymphoid follicles or percolating between lesional cells (**Fig. 6**). Lesser numbers of eosinophils, neutrophils, xanthomatous histiocytes, and osteoclast-like and Touton-like giant cells are also detected. The inflammatory component varies

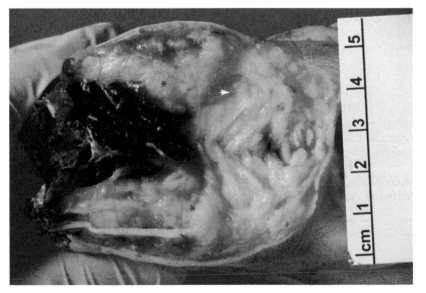

Fig. 1. Macroscopic appearance of MIFS. Bivalved specimen shows a multinodular subcutaneous mass with a glistening, tan-yellow cut surface (marked by *) and infiltrating into the fascia (*white arrow*).

Fig. 2. Scanning (*A*) and intermediate-power (*B*) magnification of MIFS commonly demonstrates a variably cellular tumor in an inflamed, fibrosclerotic stroma with scattered mucin-rich pools. (*C*). Tenosynovial involvement often manifests as myxoedematous bulbous fronds of lesional tissue.

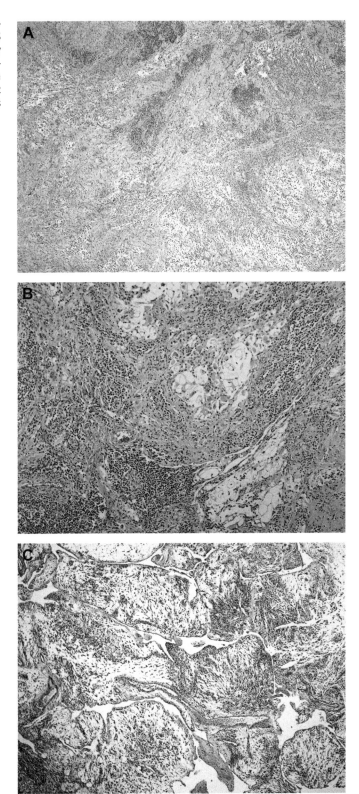

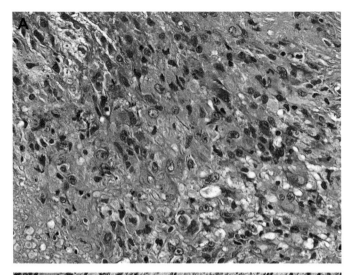

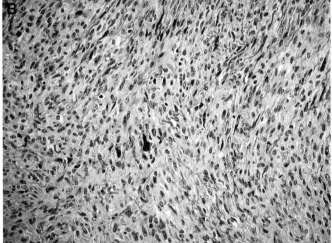

Fig. 3. Two main neoplastic cells of MIFS: (*A*). Eosinophilic epithelioid cells with distinct cell borders and vesicular nuclei with conspicuous nucleoli. Note interstitial mucin separating cells (upper left) (*B*). Mildly atypical plump spindle cells.

in density. In some tumors, dense inflammation masks lesional cells, potentially leading to a misdiagnosis of an inflammatory or lymphomatous process.

- The fibrosclerotic collagen typically forms hyalinized bulbous fronds or bands with granulation tissue-like vasculature and a paucity of inflammatory and neoplastic cells (**Fig. 7**).

Other histologic features observed in conventional MIFS include a low mitotic count (1–2 mitoses per 10 high-power fields with an average of about 3 mitoses per 50 high-power fields)[5,6] and focal necrosis.[1,2,5] Hemosiderin and/or fibrin deposits were found in over 50% of tumors in one large case study.[5]

Histology of recurrent and metastatic lesions either resembles the primary or exhibits an increased number of atypical cells mimicking a higher-grade sarcoma.[1,5]

Three tumors are currently considered potential variants of MIFS.

1. High-grade examples of MIFS demonstrate cellular foci of highly pleomorphic cells blending with conventional MIFS or transitioning abruptly to form a discrete high-grade sarcoma ("dedifferentiated MIFS"). These high-grade areas exhibit increased mitotic activity including atypical mitotic figures, tumoral necrosis, and concentrated, branching capillary or thick-walled arcuate (sarcoma-like) vasculature (**Fig. 8**).[5,13] This variant has a propensity for non-acral sites[12,13] and tends to achieve a large size.[13] Presence of "hallmark" cells of MIFS and emperipolesis assist in recognizing these lesions as MIFS variants.[13]

2. Hybrid tumors featuring MIFS-like areas and a component of relatively bland spindle cells infiltrating fat with hemosiderin deposition (hybrid

Fig. 4. "Hallmark" cells of MIFS. (*A*). RS-like cells are characterized by abundant deeply eosinophilic cytoplasm and an irregularly contoured large nucleus with vesicular chromatin and a viral inclusion-like eosinophilic macronucleolus. (*B*). RS-like variant possessing smudgy heterochromatin and resembling a mummified RS cell. (*C*). Pseudolipoblasts have pleomorphic nuclei and abundant cytoplasm distended by mucin-filled vacuoles.

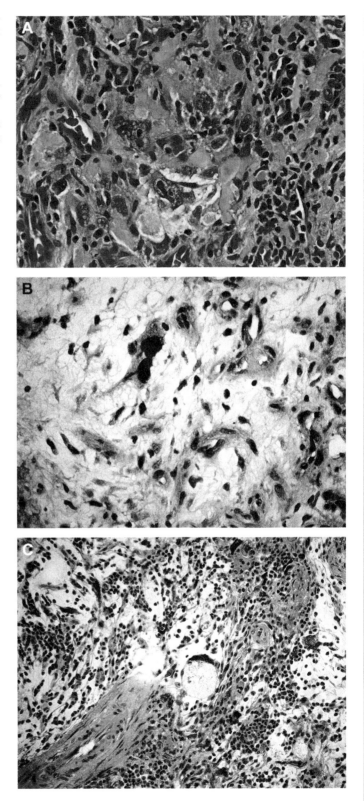

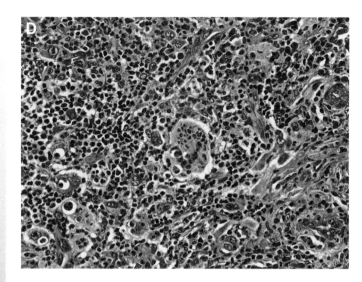

Fig. 4. (*D*). Lesional cells exhibiting emperipolesis are common but usually sparse in number.

MIFS and hemosiderotic fibrolipomatous tumor [HFLT]) have been described.[5,14–20] Recent molecular studies, however, provide an alternative explanation for this purported mixed phenotype (see later in discussion). A hybrid MIFS and pleomorphic hyalinizing angiectatic tumor (PHAT) featuring conventional or high-grade MIFS with ectatic vessels and associated intra- and extraluminal fibrin has also been described.[5,13,21] The possibility that PHAT-like changes are secondary to vascular insufficiency in a MIFS has been entertained.[5,13,21]

Indeed, the rare phenomenon of PHAT recurring as myxofibrosarcoma may represent progression of a conventional MIFS with PHAT-like vascular changes to a high-grade MIFS.[13,21]

3. Recently, a "nodular necrotizing" variant featuring centrally necrotic tumor nodules composed of epithelioid cells, numerous RS-like cells, and cells exhibiting emperipolesis has been described (**Fig. 9**). Unlike conventional MIFS, myxoid areas are sparse or absent and pseudolipoblasts are generally not found.[22]

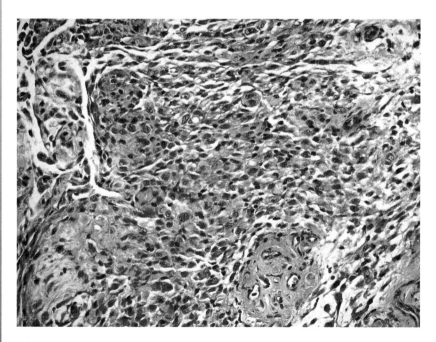

Fig. 5. Mucin-rich pools harboring trabeculae of loosely cohesive lesional cells separated by intercellular mucin.

Fig. 6. The inflammatory component of MIFS varies in density, occasionally masking lesional cells, and consists mainly of lymphocytes and plasma cells.

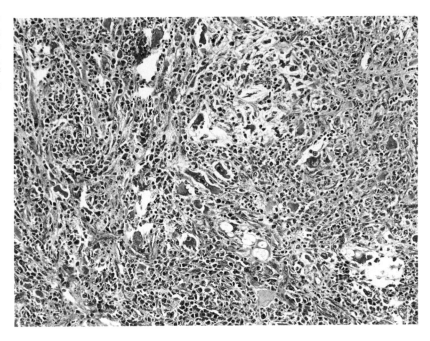

A subsequent study of malignant epithelioid neoplasms with *MAML2* rearrangements detailed 2 cases with a *YAP1* partner and overlapping features with the "nodular necrotizing" variant.[23]

ANCILLARY STUDIES

Currently, cyclin D1, PRAME, Factor XIIIa, and CD10 have shown high sensitivity, but low specificity, diffusely marking tumor cells in nearly all tumors tested. The former 2 immunomarkers assist in identifying emperipolesis as engulfed inflammatory cell are negative.[6,13,22,24] Membranous D2-40 positivity is found in over 60% of tumors with the majority of lesional cells staining positive.[5,6,24] Epithelial membrane antigen was reported as focally expressed in 72% and EGFR in 88% of cases in one study.[25] Diffuse positivity for the histiocyte marker CD163 was documented

Fig. 7. Paucicellular fibrosclerotic stroma with granulation tissue-like vasculature.

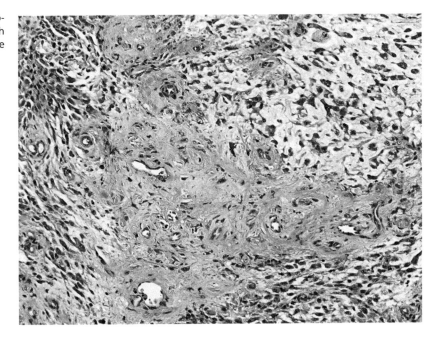

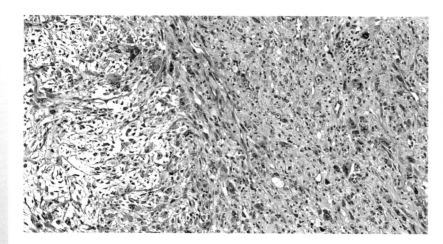

Fig. 8. High-grade MIFS shows areas of hypercellularity, nuclear pleomorphism, and increased mitotic activity, not unlike an undifferentiated pleomorphic sarcoma. (Photomicrograph courtesy of Dr. Michal Michal)

in all 16 tumors tested in one study.[25] However, CD68 (KP1), a lysozyme marker that also highlights histiocytes, was found in only a minority of tumor cells in a larger number of cases.[2,5,6,26]

Thus, it is likely that reported CD163 positivity reflects the staining of intralesional histiocytes. CD34, keratin (mainly pan-keratin AE1/3), muscle actins, and desmin expression is focal and

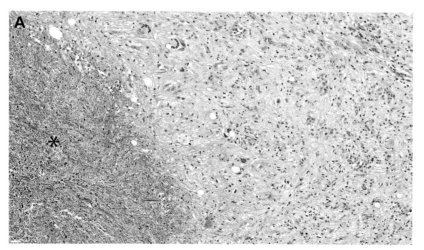

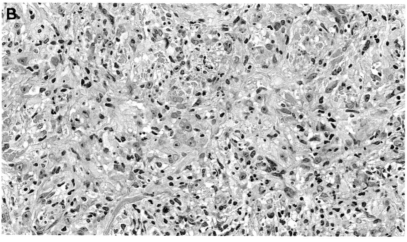

Fig. 9. (*A, B*) Nodular necrotizing MIFS features nodules with central necrosis (marked by *) surrounded by epithelioid cells, spindle cells, RS-like cells, and cells with emperipolesis. (Photomicrograph courtesy of Dr. Raul Perret)

generally found in less than 50% of tumors tested.[2,5,6,8,22,24–26]

Three main molecular events have been detected in conventional MIFS along with other additional complex karyotypes.[15,27,28] However, they are all nonspecific.

Amplification of VGLL3 on 3p11-12 in a supernumerary ring chromosome is reported in approximately 47% of MIFS evaluated[6,15,24,27,29,30] and represents the most frequent molecular aberration currently detected in MIFS. VGLL3 amplification may coexist with either BRAF mutation or t(1;10) translocation. In cases lacking VGLL3 amplification, a SEC23IP::VGLL3 or a TEAD1::MRTFB rearrangement has been reported.[24] VGLL3 is a cofactor for the TEAD family of transcriptional factors and genetic alterations in VGLL3 are believed to dysregulate TEAD target genes and result in cell proliferation.[31]

A t(1;10) with breakpoints found around OGA on 10q24 and TGFBR3 on 1p22 or rearrangements of either TGFBR3 or OGA are documented in approximately 16% of pure MIFS tested.[6,15,19,20,24,27,30] As pure HFLT[15,20,27] and purported examples of hybrid MIFS-HFLT tumors exhibit substantially higher frequencies of these translocations compared with pure MIFS,[20] some believe that HFLT and MIFS are separate entities and examples of so-called "hybrid MIFS-HFLT"[14–16,32] and cases of HFLT recurring as a higher-grade sarcoma[17,19,33] may actually represent progression of HFLT to a myxoid sarcoma demonstrating features reminiscent of MIFS.[20] Deep sequencing has shown that the t(1;10) breakpoints vary, resulting in inconsistent rearrangements.[30] Therefore, cases with either TGFBR3 or OGA rearrangement by FISH may have a t(1;10) with gene breakpoints not detected by the conventional probes used. As the t(1;10) fusion partners are transcribed in different directions, no functional fusion transcript or protein is detected. Instead, the translocation leads to the upregulation of NPM3 and FGF8 near OGA[27] with FGF8 in particular appearing to play a role in the tumor's pathogenesis.[27,30]

BRAF fusions, and less often amplification, are found in approximately 10% of MIFS including the "nodular necrotizing" variant, are mutually exclusive of t(1;10), and currently have not been detected in either pure HFLT or hybrid HFLT-MIFS and HFLT-PHAT tumors.[6,24,29,30] BRAF-mutated MIFS shows a predilection for acral sites.[29] The fusion partners include ZNF335,[6] TOM1L2,[29] SND1,[24] and ROBO1.[30]

A YAP1::MAML2 fusion was detected in 3 out of 7 cases (43%) of the nodular necrotizing variant by RNA sequencing, while none of the cases demonstrated VGLL3 amplification.[22]

DIFFERENTIAL DIAGNOSIS

HEMOSIDEROTIC FIBROLIPOMATOUS TUMOR (HFLT) AND PLEOMORPHIC HYALINIZING ANGIECTATIC TUMOR (PHAT)

- The histogenetic relationship between HFLT, PHAT and MIFS has been a matter of continuing debate, complicated by partially shared histologic and immunohistochemical features and a lack of specific molecular aberrations (Table 1).[15,21,27,34,35] Clinically, both PHAT and HFLT have a more restricted distribution than MIFS, arising almost exclusively in the superficial soft tissues of the foot and ankle. Nearly one-half of patients with HFLT relate a history of prior trauma or vasculopathy.[34,36]
- HFLT consists of mildly atypical, spindled cells with intracytoplasmic hemosiderin within a fibromyxoid stroma, osteoclast-like giant cells, hemosiderin-laden macrophages, and a scant lymphoplasmacytic infiltrate. Variably sized fascicles of tumor cells characteristically proliferate between lobules of adipose tissue.[36,37]
- PHAT features scattered clusters of ectatic thin-walled vessels with intraluminal thrombi and fibrin, surrounding fibrin-like hyaline material, and a mixed inflammatory infiltrate. The lesional element consists of cytologically bland spindled cells arranged in sheets and fascicles. A minor population of pleomorphic cells with cytoplasmic hemosiderin and hyperchromatic nuclei often harboring intranuclear pseudoinclusions, but exhibiting low mitotic activity, are characteristic.[38,39] Cells with features overlapping with RS-like cells or pseudolipoblasts of MIFS are occasionally identified.[34] In nearly 50% of reported cases, bland spindle cells with associated hemosiderin infiltrate subcutaneous adipose tissue at the periphery of PHAT. This HFLT-like change is termed "early PHAT."[39]

TENOSYNOVIAL GIANT CELL TUMOR

- Localized TSGCTs typically involve the tenosynovium of the fingers as do many examples of MIFS (Table 1). TSGCTs are composed of small neoplastic epithelioid cells, histiocytes (± xanthomatous change), osteoclast-like giant cells, and scattered inflammatory cells.[40] The neoplastic cell has well-defined cell borders often with a cytoplasmic rim of hemosiderin and a rounded vesicular nucleus with a conspicuous nucleolus. This cell marks with

Table 1
Mesenchymal tumors in the differential diagnosis of MIFS: key clinical and pathologic differences

Parameters Compared with MIFS	PHAT	HFLT	Tenosynovial Giant Cell Tumor	Myxofibrosarcoma	Superficial CD34 +
Peak age	NA	NA	Early to middle-age adulthood	Middle to late-age adulthood	NA
Common Location/Depth	Foot and ankles/NA	Dorsal foot and ankle/NA	Digits (most common location of localized variant), knee, hip, ankle/Deep (articular/periarticular)	Appendicular soft tissue (uncommon in acral sites)/Superficial > Deep	Proximal lower extremities (uncommon in acral sites)/NA
IHC/Molecular (lesional cells)	More diffuse CD34 (>80% cases); no *BRAF* mutations	More diffuse CD34 (>80% cases); no *BRAF* mutations	Clusterin (5)	NA	CADM3 and WT1, more diffuse CD34 (6)
Histology	Vascular and "early PHAT" changes; (−) paucicellular fibrosclerotic stroma	Infiltration of subcutaneous fat; (−) pseudolipoblasts, RS-like cells, or mixed inflammatory infiltrate	(−) RS-like cells, pseudolipoblasts, or myxoid areas	Prominent branching/curvilinear vessels, diffusely myxoid stroma and less inflammation; high-grade MIFS and myxofibrosarcoma may have solid cellular foci of pleomorphic cells	Uniform growth pattern and greater degree of pleomorphism; (−) paucicellular fibrosclerotic stroma and myxoid pools/lakes

Abbreviations: (−), lack of; >, more than; HFLT, hemosiderotic fibrolipomatous tumor; IHC, immunohistochemistry; MIFS, myxoinflammatory fibroblastic sarcoma; NA, parameter does not assist in the differential diagnosis; PHAT, pleomorphic hyalinizing angiectatic tumor; RS, Reed-Sternberg; SUPERFICIAL CD34+- Superficial CD34-positive fibroblastic tumor.

D2-40 and clusterin in keeping with its purported synovial cell-type differentiation.[41]

MYXOFIBROSARCOMA

- MFS typically presents as a slow-growing mass in the superficial and slightly less often deep soft tissue of lower extremities, followed by the upper extremities and trunk (**Table 1**). Morphologically, MFS is characterized by ill-defined, extensively myxoid nodules populated by atypical spindled and stellate cells, pseudolipoblasts, and associated curvilinear, thick-walled and branching vessels.[42]

SUPERFICIAL CD34-POSITIVE FIBROBLASTIC TUMOR

- SCD34FT occurs in the superficial soft tissues of the lower extremities, followed by the upper extremities and trunk. Microscopically, it is comprised of highly pleomorphic plump spindled and epithelioid cells growing in fascicular and storiform arrays. The cells have abundant eosinophilic glassy, coarsely granular, or less often vacuolated (lipoblast-like) or fibrillary cytoplasm. The mitotic count is disproportionally low for the degree of pleomorphism. A mixed inflammatory infiltrate and an accentuated vascular component are often present.[43] SCD34FT shows strong and diffuse expression of CD34 and CADM3, a protein upregulated due to *PRDM10* gene rearrangements.[44] Nuclear immunoreactivity for WT-1 is reported in 75% of cases.[44] Keratin and desmin may also be focally positive by immunohistochemistry.

HEMATOPOIETIC NEOPLASMS

Soft Tissue Rosai-Dorfman Disease

Soft tissue RDD typically involves superficial soft tissue and features a prominent lymphoplasmacytic infiltrate and large epithelioid histiocytes exhibiting emperipolesis. Unlike MIFS, RDD lacks the mucin deposition and "hallmark" cells of MIFS, and the spindled and epithelioid histiocytes of RDD express S100 protein and OCT2.[45]

Hodgkin Lymphoma and Extranodal Anaplastic Large Cell Lymphoma

Both MIFS and eALCL involve superficial soft tissue, while classic HL arises in deeper tissue. Epithelioid cells with RS-like nuclei and a dense inflammatory background are shared by both MIFS and HL. The "hallmark" cell of ALCL possesses eosinophilic cytoplasm, a perinuclear "hof", and a reniform nucleus with vesicular chromatin and a conspicuous nucleolus. True RS cells are immunopositive for PAX5, CD15 and CD30, while ALCL cells stain for CD30 and may express ALK and T-lymphocyte markers.

PROGNOSIS

- The reported recurrence rate for conventional MIFS is about 27%[4,5,11] with nearly 12% of patients experiencing 2 or more recurrences.[4,5] The median time to recurrence is 14 to 15 months.[4,5] Incomplete surgical excision with positive surgical margins[5] and short symptom duration (6 months or less)[4] have been statistically correlated with recurrence. In the initial study, all 6 individuals with the "nodular necrotizing" variant showed no evidence of recurrence or metastasis after at least a 6-month follow-up interval.
- Metastases are documented in approximately 2% of conventional MIFS, usually after local recurrence.[4,26,46] Metastatic sites are most commonly regional lymph nodes and lung.[1,2,4–6,13] MIFS-related death is extremely rare.[4]
- Although no histologic feature absolutely predicts aggressive behavior in MIFS, the reported recurrence rate in tumors exhibiting high-grade histologic features with at least 6 months of follow-up is 56% and the metastatic rate is 33%.[5,12,13]
- Wide local surgical excision ensuring negative surgical margins is the treatment of choice. One study reported no recurrence or metastases in 13 patients with MIFS treated initially with surgery and preoperative radiation, including 5 individuals with positive surgical margins (4 of which were given postoperative radiation) after a median follow-up interval of over 24 months.[47] Experience with Mohs surgery is limited.[48,49]

SUMMARY

The conventional MIFS is a low-grade fibroblastic sarcoma that predilects to the superficial soft tissues of the distal extremity. The tumor is composed of neoplastic plump spindled and epithelioid cells, inflammatory infiltrates, and mucin deposits in a fibrosclerotic stroma. Cells characteristic of the entity are RS-like epithelioid cells, pleomorphic pseudolipoblasts, and cells exhibiting emperipolesis. These cells assist in confirming the diagnosis in cases exhibiting high-grade or sarcomatous features. Immunohistochemistry plays a limited diagnostic role and MIFS has recurrent non-specific molecular aberrations, many of which are shared by HFLT and PHAT. Wide local surgical excision is the treatment of choice. Recurrence is not uncommon and likely related to the completeness of initial excision and a short duration of presenting symptoms. Metastatic spread is rare in classic MIFS but is documented more often in tumors exhibiting high-grade histologic features.

CLINICS CARE POINTS

- MIFS is composed of neoplastic epithelioid and spindled cells, a variable inflammatory infiltrate, and a fibrosclerotic stroma punctuated by mucin deposits.

- Cellular elements characteristic of MIFS include RS-like cells, pleomorphic pseudolipoblasts, and cells exhibiting emperipolesis.

- Cyclin D1, CD10, Factor XIIIa, and PRAME are relatively sensitive but nonspecific immunomarkers.

- *VGLL3* amplification, t(1;10), and/or *BRAF* mutations occur in a significant minority of tumors, but are nonspecific.

- MIFS has locally recurrent potential if incompletely excised, but low risk for metastasis. Tumors exhibiting high-grade histologic features demonstrate higher rates of recurrence and metastasis.

REFERENCES

1. Meis-Kindblom JM, Kindblom LG. Acral myxoinflammatory fibroblastic sarcoma: a low-grade tumor of the hands and feet. Am J Surg Pathol 1998;22: 911–24.

2. Montgomery EA, Devaney KO, Giordano TJ, et al. Inflammatory myxohyaline tumor of distal extremities with virocyte or Reed-Sternberg-like cells: a distinctive lesion with features simulating inflammatory conditions, Hodgkin's disease, and various sarcomas. Mod Pathol 1998;11:384–91.

3. Michal M. Inflammatory myxoid tumor of the soft parts with bizarre giant cells. Pathol Res Pract 1998;194: 529–33.

4. Lombardi R, Jovine E, Zanini N, et al. A case of lung metastasis in myxoinflammatory fibroblastic sarcoma: analytical review of one hundred and thirty eight cases. Int Orthop 2013;37:2429–36.

5. Laskin WB, Fetsch JF, Miettinen M. Myxoinflammatory fibroblastic sarcoma: a clinicopathologic analysis of 104 cases, with emphasis on predictors of outcome. Am J Surg Pathol 2014;38:1–12.

6. Suster D, Michal M, Huang H, et al. Myxoinflammatory fibroblastic sarcoma: an immunohistochemical and molecular genetic study of 73 cases. Mod Pathol 2020;33:2520–33.

7. Alaggio R, Coffin CM, Dall'igna P, et al. Myxoinflammatory fibroblastic sarcoma: report of a case and review of the literature. Pediatr Dev Pathol 2012;15:254–8.

8. Weiss VL, Antonescu CR, Alaggio R, et al. Myxoinflammatory fibroblastic sarcoma in children and adolescents: clinicopathologic aspects of a rare neoplasm. Pediatr Dev Pathol 2013;16:425–31.

9. Jain E, Kini L, Alaggio R, et al. Myxoinflammatory fibroblastic sarcoma of eyeball in an infant: a rare presentation. Int J Surg Pathol 2020;28:306–9.

10. Tateishi U, Hasegawa T, Nojima T, et al. MRI features of extraskeletal myxoid chondrosarcoma. Skeletal Radiol 2006;35:27–33.

11. Kumar R, Lefkowitz RA, Neto AD. Myxoinflammatory fibroblastic sarcoma: clinical, imaging, management and outcome in 29 patients. J Comput Assist Tomogr 2017;41:104–15.

12. Gaetke-Udager K, Yablon CM, Lucas DR, et al. Myxoinflammatory fibroblastic sarcoma: spectrum of disease and imaging presentation. Skeletal Radiol 2016;45:347–56.

13. Michal M, Kazakov DV, Hadravsky L, et al. High-grade myxoinflammatory fibroblastic sarcoma: a report of 23 cases. Ann Diagn Pathol 2015;19:157–63.

14. Elco CP, Marino-Enriquez A, Abraham JA, et al. Hybrid myxoinflammatory fibroblastic sarcoma/hemosiderotic fibrolipomatous tumor: report of a case providing further evidence for a pathogenetic link. Am J Surg Pathol 2010;34:1723–7.

15. Antonescu CR, Zhang L, Nielsen GP, et al. Consistent t(1;10) with rearrangements of TGFBR3 and MGEA5 in both myxoinflammatory fibroblastic sarcoma and hemosiderotic fibrolipomatous tumor. Genes Chromosomes Cancer 2011;50:757–64.

16. Rekhi B, Adamane S. Myxoinflammatory fibroblastic sarcoma with areas resembling hemosiderotic fibrolipomatous tumor: a rare case indicating proximity between the two tumors. Indian J Pathol Microbiol 2014;57:647–8.

17. O'Driscoll D, Athanasian E, Hameed M, et al. Radiological imaging features and clinicopathological correlation of hemosiderotic fibrolipomatous tumor: experience in a single tertiary cancer center. Skeletal Radiol 2015;44:641–8.

18. Hallin M, Miki Y, Hayes AJ, et al. Acral myxoinflammatory fibroblastic sarcoma with hybrid features of hemosiderotic fibrolipomatous tumor occurring 10 years after renal transplantation. Rare Tumors 2018;10, 2036361318782626.

19. Carter JM, Sukov WR, Montgomery E, et al. TGFBR3 and MGEA5 rearrangements in pleomorphic hyalinizing angiectatic tumors and the spectrum of related neoplasms. Am J Surg Pathol 2014;38:1182–992.

20. Zreik RT, Carter JM, Sukov WR, et al. TGFBR3 and MGEA5 rearrangements are much more common in "hybrid" hemosiderotic fibrolipomatous tumor-myxoinflammatory fibroblastic sarcomas than in classical myxoinflammatory fibroblastic sarcomas: a morphological and fluorescence in situ hybridization study. Hum Pathol 2016;53:14–24.

21. Michal M, Kazakov DV, Hadravsky L, et al. Pleomorphic hyalinizing angiectatic tumor revisited: all tumors manifest typical morphologic features of myxoinflammatory fibroblastic sarcoma, further suggesting 2 morphologic variants of a single entity. Ann Diagn Pathol 2016;20:40–3.

22. Perret R, Tallegas M, Velasco V, et al. Recurrent YAP1::MAML2 fusions in "nodular necrotizing" variants of myxoinflammatory fibroblastic sarcoma: a comprehensive study of 7 cases. Mod Pathol 2022;35:1398–404.

23. Dermawan JK, DiNapoli SE, Sukhadia P, et al. Malignant undifferentiated epithelioid neoplasms with MAML2 rearrangements: A clinicopathologic study of seven cases demonstrating a heterogenous entity. Genes Chromosomes Cancer 2023;62:191–201.

24. Klubickova N, Agaimy A, Hajkova V, et al. RNA-sequencing of myxoinflammatory fibroblastic sarcomas reveals a novel SND1::BRAF fusion and 3 different molecular aberrations with the potential to upregulate the TEAD1 gene including SEC23IP::VGLL3 and TEAD1::MRTFB gene fusions. Virchows Arch 2022;481:613–20.

25. Kovarik CL, Barrett T, Auerbach A, et al. Acral myxoinflammatory fibroblastic sarcoma: case series and immunohistochemical analysis. J Cutan Pathol 2008;35:192–6.

26. Sakaki M, Hirokawa M, Wakatsuki S, et al. Acral myxoinflammatory fibroblastic sarcoma: a report of five cases and review of the literature. Virchows Arch 2003;442:25–30.

27. Hallor KH, Sciot R, Staaf J, et al. Two genetic pathways, t(1;10) and amplification of 3p11-12, in myxoinflammatory fibroblastic sarcoma, haemosiderotic fibrolipomatous tumour, and morphologically similar lesions. J Pathol 2009;217:716–27.

28. Gonzalez-Campora R, Rios-Martin JJ, Solorzano-Amoretti A, et al. Fine needle aspiration cytology of an acral myxoinflammatory fibroblastic sarcoma: case report with cytological and cytogenetic findings. Cytopathology 2008;19:118–23.

29. Kao YC, Ranucci V, Zhang L, et al. Recurrent BRAF gene rearrangements in myxoinflammatory fibroblastic sarcomas, but not hemosiderotic fibrolipomatous tumors. Am J Surg Pathol 2017;41:1456–65.

30. Arbajian E, Hofvander J, Magnusson L, et al. Deep sequencing of myxoinflammatory fibroblastic sarcoma. Genes Chromosomes Cancer 2020;59:309–17.

31. Yamaguchi N. Multiple roles of vestigial-like family members in tumor development. Front Oncol 2020;10:1266.

32. Marusic Z, Cengic T, Dzombeta T, et al. Hybrid myxoinflammatory fibroblastic sarcoma/hemosiderotic fibrolipomatous tumor of the ankle following repeated trauma. Pathol Int 2014;64:195–7.

33. Solomon DA, Antonescu CR, Link TM, et al. Hemosiderotic fibrolipomatous tumor, not an entirely benign entity. Am J Surg Pathol 2013;37:1627–30.

34. Liu H, Sukov WR, Ro JY. The t(1;10)(p22;q24) TGFBR3/MGEA5 translocation in pleomorphic hyalinizing angiectatic tumor, myxoinflammatory fibroblastic sarcoma, and hemosiderotic fibrolipomatous tumor. Arch Pathol Lab Med 2019;143:212–21.

35. Boland JM, Folpe AL. Hemosiderotic fibrolipomatous tumor, pleomorphic hyalinizing angiectatic tumor, and myxoinflammatory fibroblastic sarcoma: related or not? Adv Anat Pathol 2017;24:268–77.

36. Marshall-Taylor C, Fanburg-Smith JC. Hemosiderotic fibrohistiocytic lipomatous lesion: ten cases of a previously undescribed fatty lesion of the foot/ankle. Mod Pathol 2000;13:1192–9.

37. Browne TJ, Fletcher CD. Haemosiderotic fibrolipomatous tumour (so-called haemosiderotic fibrohistiocytic lipomatous tumour): analysis of 13 new cases in support of a distinct entity. Histopathology 2006;48:453–61.

38. Smith ME, Fisher C, Weiss SW. Pleomorphic hyalinizing angiectatic tumor of soft parts. A low-grade neoplasm resembling neurilemoma. Am J Surg Pathol 1996;20:21–9.

39. Folpe AL, Weiss SW. Pleomorphic hyalinizing angiectatic tumor: analysis of 41 cases supporting evolution from a distinctive precursor lesion. Am J Surg Pathol 2004;28:1417–25.

40. Rao AS, Vigorita VJ. Pigmented villonodular synovitis (giant-cell tumor of the tendon sheath and synovial membrane). A review of eighty-one cases. J Bone Joint Surg Am 1984;66:76–94.

41. Boland JM, Folpe AL, Hornick JL, et al. Clusterin is expressed in normal synoviocytes and in tenosynovial giant cell tumors of localized and diffuse types: diagnostic and histogenetic implications. Am J Surg Pathol 2009;33:1225–9.

42. Angervall L, Kindblom LG, Merck C, et al. A study of 30 cases. Acta Pathol Microbiol Scand 1977;85A:127–40.

43. Carter JM, Weiss SW, Linos K, et al. Superficial CD34-positive fibroblastic tumor: report of 18 cases of a distinctive low-grade mesenchymal neoplasm of intermediate (borderline) malignancy. Mod Pathol 2014;27:294–302.

44. Anderson WJ, Mertens F, Marino-Enriquez A, et al. Superficial CD34-positive fibroblastic tumor: a clinicopathologic, immunohistochemical, and molecular

study of 59 cases. Am J Surg Pathol 2022;46: 1329–39.

45. Ravindran A, Goyal G, Go RS, et al. Mayo Clinic Histiocytosis Working G. Rosai-Dorfman disease displays a unique monocyte-macrophage phenotype characterized by expression of OCT2. Am J Surg Pathol 2021;45:35–44.

46. Hassanein AM, Atkinson SP, Al-Quran SZ, et al. Acral myxoinflammatory fibroblastic sarcomas: are they all low-grade neoplasms? J Cutan Pathol 2008;35:186–91.

47. Tejwani A, Kobayashi W, Chen YL, et al. Management of acral myxoinflammatory fibroblastic sarcoma. Cancer 2010;116:5733–9.

48. D'Elia MLN, Park KK, Weiss E. Acral myxoinflammatory fibroblastic sarcoma: report of a case and treatment with mohs micrographic surgery. J Clin Aesthet Dermatol 2020;13:35–7.

49. Tivoli YA, Thomas JA, Chen AF, et al. Acral myxoinflammatory fibroblastic sarcoma successfully treated using Mohs micrographic surgery. Dermatol Surg 2013;39:1709–11.

Atypical Spindle Cell/ Pleomorphic Lipomatous Tumor

Amir Qorbani, MD*, Andrew Horvai, MD, PhD

KEYWORDS

- Soft tissue • Atypical spindle cell lipomatous tumor • Spindle cell lipoma • Liposarcoma

---

Key points

- Atypical spindle cell/pleomorphic lipomatous tumor (ASCPLT) chiefly affects middle-aged adults, arising in the subcutis of the extremities.
- Microscopically, ASCPLT consists of a lipogenic neoplasm with atypical spindled and/or pleomorphic cells and infiltrative borders.
- Ancillary tests to support the diagnosis of ASCPLT include CD34 immunopositivity, loss of Rb expression or *RB1* gene deletion, and lack of *MDM2* amplification or *DDIT3* rearrangement.
- Behavior is generally benign with up to ~10-15% local recurrence and no metastasis.

ABSTRACT

Atypical spindle cell/pleomorphic lipomatous tumor (ASCPLT) is a rare soft tissue neoplasm, commonly arising in the subcutis (more common than deep soft tissue) of limbs and limb girdles during mid-adulthood. ASCPLT is histologically a lipogenic neoplasm with ill-defined margins composed of a variable amount of spindle to pleomorphic/multinucleated cells within a fibromyxoid stroma. ASCPLTs lack *MDM2* amplification, but a large subset show *RB1* deletion and variable expression of CD34. Though initially thought to be the malignant form of spindle cell lipoma, ASCPLTs are benign with local recurrences (~10-15%) and no well-documented dedifferentiation or metastasis.

OVERVIEW

Atypical spindle cell/pleomorphic lipomatous tumor (ASCPLT) was originally considered as an uncommon variant of atypical lipomatous tumor/well-differentiated liposarcoma, as it was reflected in the 3rd and 4th edition of the WHO Classification of Tumours of Soft Tissue and Bone.[1,2] In 1994, Dei Tos and colleagues[3] proposed the term "spindle cell liposarcoma" as a separate entity based on a study of 6 cases, which were primarily located in the subcutis of the shoulder, and composed of bland spindle cells arranged in whorls and fascicles. In 2010, Mentzel and colleagues[4] described these tumors as the atypical counterpart of spindle cell lipoma, based on a clinicopathologic, immunohistochemical, and molecular analysis of 6 cases, which revealed indolent clinical behavior, variable CD34 immunoreactivity, presence of *RB1* gene deletion, and lack of *MDM2* amplification. In 2013, Deyrup and colleagues[5] described these tumors as "fibrosarcoma-like lipomatous neoplasms," which were composed of nodules of differentiated fibroblastic cells showing varying degrees of lipoblastic differentiation reminiscent of the early stages of embryonic fat development.

Pathology, University of California, 1825 4th Street, Room M2369, Box 4066, San Francisco, CA 94158-4066, USA
* Corresponding author.
E-mail address: Amir.Qorbani@ucsf.edu

Surgical Pathology 17 (2024) 97–104
https://doi.org/10.1016/j.path.2023.07.004

In 2014, Creytens and colleagues[6] described not only *RB1* deletion, but also the deletion of flanking genes *ITM2B*, *RCBTB2*, and *DLEU1*, and classified the tumors as "atypical spindle cell lipoma." In 2017, Mariño-Enriquez and colleagues.[7] coined the term "atypical spindle cell lipomatous tumor (ASCLT)" based on the clinicopathologic characterization of 232 cases. They defined ASCLT as a lipogenic neoplasm with (1) a tendency to arise in distal extremities, (2) histologic resemblance to spindle cell lipoma with increased cellularity, mild-to-moderate nuclear atypia/hyperchromasia and (3) a generally benign behavior. Subsequent reports[8,9] have been in agreement with the clinicopathologic definition of ASCLT proposed by Mariño-Enriquez and colleagues.[7] In 2020, atypical spindle cell/pleomorphic lipomatous tumors were classified as a separate entity by the 5th edition WHO Classification of Tumours of Soft Tissue and Bone.[10] The more recently proposed diagnoses of "anisometric cell lipoma," and "dysplastic lipoma"[11–13] may also represent variants of ASCPLT.[10]

GROSS FEATURES

Grossly, atypical spindle cell/pleomorphic lipomatous tumor (ASCPLT) is usually an ill-defined nodular or multinodular mass, ranging from 0.5 to 28 cm with median size of 5-8.5 cm[7] The cut surface varies from yellow to white-gray, to myxoid, depending on the relative amount of adipocytic and spindle cell components and myxoid stroma, respectively. Unlike spindle cell lipoma, ASCPLT can rarely involve fascia and deeper soft tissues.

MICROSCOPIC FEATURES

ASCPLT is characterized by mature adipose tissue with variability in adipocyte size, lipoblasts, relatively uniform plump bipolar spindle cells, and floret-like multinucleated giant cells in a collagenous and/or myxoid matrix. The collagen may be arranged in thick bundles forming a so-called "ropy" pattern. The ratio of these components can vary dramatically between and even within

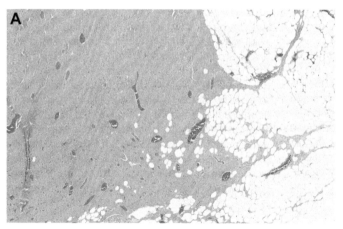
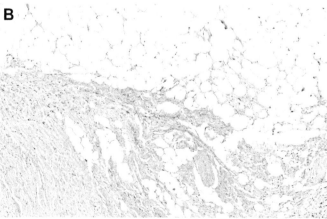

Fig. 1. ASCPLT with ill-defined borders: (*A*). Atypical spindle cell lipomatous tumor at low magnification (40x original magnification): H&E-stained section shows a spindle cell proliferation with infiltrating borders. (*B*). Atypical pleomorphic lipomatous tumor at low magnification (100x original magnification): H&E-stained section show a pleomorphic spindle cell proliferation with infiltrating borders.

Fig. 2. Cytological features of ASCPLT: (*A*). Atypical spindle cell lipomatous tumor at high magnification (400x original magnification): H&E-stained section shows spindle cells with low to moderate atypia within a collagenous stroma. (*B*). Atypical pleomorphic lipomatous tumor at high magnification (400x magnification): H&E-stained section shows a lipogenic neoplasm with spindle to pleomorphic cells, atypical lipoblasts, and scattered multinuclear cells.

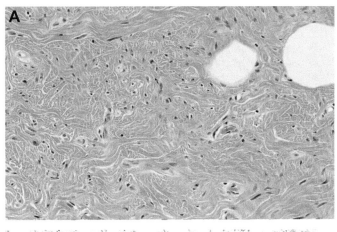

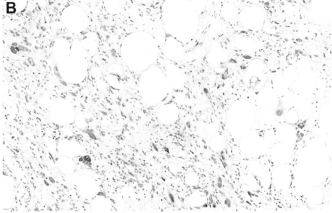

tumors and thus ASCPLT bears resemblance to spindle cell lipoma. Unlike spindle cell lipoma, however, ASCPLT shows one or more of the following features: infiltrating margins (**Fig. 1**), pleomorphic lipoblasts, pleomorphic and/or bizarre multinucleated cells, nuclear atypia and/or hyperchromasia in the spindle cells (**Fig. 2**). Mitotic activity is more conspicuous than in spindle cell lipoma, but atypical mitoses are unusual (**Fig. 3**). Coagulative tumor necrosis is typically absent although fat necrosis with foamy macrophages may be present.

Although a range of lipogenic differentiation and cellularity exists in ASCPLT,[3–8] most tumors fall into one of the 2 subtypes.[7] At one end of the spectrum, the tumors are predominantly lipogenic with myxoid stroma and scant spindle cells, a subset of which show nuclear atypia and/or hyperchromasia (**Fig. 4A**). This subset has a predilection for the distal extremities.[6–8] Conversely, the cellular variant contains predominantly atypical spindle cells and

lipoblasts, but only scant stroma or adipose tissue.[5–7] (**Fig. 4B**) The cellular variant appears to arise in more proximal locations.[5] Mitotic figures can be seen, but are mostly scarce.[8] Mast cells, a nonspecific finding, may be present in both subtypes. ASCPLT lacks a specific vascular pattern.

ANCILLARY DIAGNOSTIC STUDIES

In 50-70% of cases, the tumor cells show loss of Rb immunoexpression.[7–9] (**Fig. 5**) Expression of CD34 (**Fig. 6**), S100, and desmin has been reported in a subset of cases (approximately 60%, 40%, and 20%, respectively).[7] The loss of Rb protein expression appears to be driven by the deletion of chromosome 13q14, encompassing the *RB1* gene, along with losses in the three nearest flanking genes *ITM2B*, *RCBTB2*, and *DLEU1*.[4,6–8] *MDM2* gene amplification on chromosome 12q13-15 is absent in ASCPLTs.[7,8] It should be noted that 13q14 loss and *RB1* gene deletion are

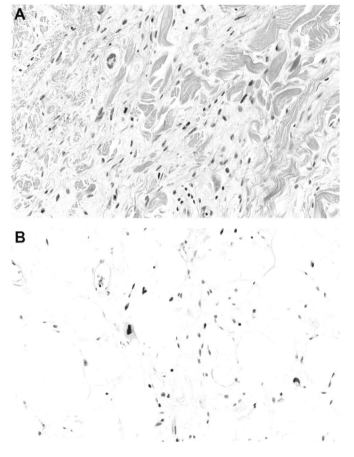

Fig. 3. Mitotic activity in ASCPLT: (*A*). Atypical spindle cell lipomatous tumor at high magnification (400x original magnification): H&E-stained section shows spindle cells with mitotic activity within a fibromyxoid stroma, ropey collagen, and scattered mast cells. (*B*). Atypical pleomorphic lipomatous tumor at high magnification (400x magnification): H&E-stained section shows a lipogenic neoplasm with scattered atypical cells and a mitotic figure.

not pathognomonic for ASCPLT (or, for that matter, spindle cell lipoma), since these alterations have been described in some forms of pleomorphic liposarcoma[14] and non-lipogenic sarcomas.[15]

DIFFERENTIAL DIAGNOSIS

The presence of spindle cells and pleomorphic cells in a lipogenic neoplasm chiefly raises three differential diagnoses.

1. *Atypical lipomatous tumor/well-differentiated liposarcoma* (ALT/WDL) demonstrates the greatest morphologic overlap with ASCPLT. Both tumors can show a range of cellularity, variably sized adipocytes, and lipoblasts. However, ALT/WDL is generally centered in deep soft tissue or retroperitoneum, is often >10 cm, and lacks the ropy collagen of ASCPLT. However, the morphologic overlap is significant, such that the detection of *MDM2* amplification or *RB1* deletion may be necessary to distinguish between ALT/WDL and ASCPLT, respectively.[7,8]

2. *Spindle cell/pleomorphic lipoma* (SCL/PL) shares many of the morphologic features of ASCPLT, especially at the fat-rich, paucicellular end of the ASCPLT spectrum. Clinically, SCL/PL has a tendency to arise in the upper back and neck region, whereas ASCPLT tends to involve the extremities, though these anatomic sites are hardly specific. Features supporting ASCPLT over SCL/PL include deep location, infiltrative borders, scattered atypical cells with bizarre nuclei, and/or atypical lipoblasts. Of note, CD34 expression and *RB1* deletion do not distinguish between SCL/PL and ASCPLT, but in the few cases studied, a more complex genetic profile may support ASCPLT.[6]

3. The distinction between *pleomorphic liposarcoma* and ASCPLT can be challenging.

Fig. 4. ASCPLT has a variable range of cellularity: (*A*). Example of hypocellular ASCPLT at high magnification (400x magnification): H&E-stained section shows a lipogenic neoplasm with scattered atypical cells, lipoblasts, and floret-type multinucleated cells within a fibromyxoid stroma. (*B*). Example of a hypercellular ASCPLT at high magnification (400x original magnification): H&E-stained section shows atypical spindle to pleomorphic cells within a fibrotic stroma. Lipogenic differentiation can be focal in the hypercellular variant of ASCPLT and is entirely absent in the region shown at this magnification.

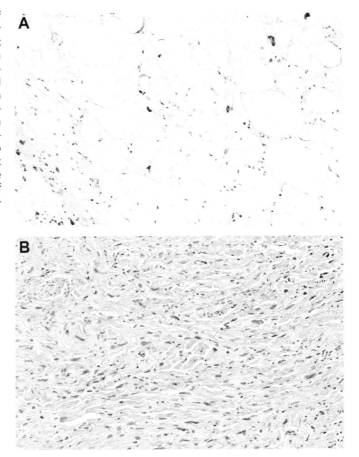

Pleomorphic liposarcoma tends to show high cellularity, diffuse, marked pleomorphism, high mitotic activity including atypical forms, coagulative tumor necrosis, and/or sheets of pleomorphic lipoblasts. These features are rare to absent in ASCPLT. In contrast, the presence of floret-like multinucleated cells and ropey collagen supports ASCPLT over pleomorphic liposarcoma.[8] CD34 may be less frequently positive in pleomorphic liposarcoma than ASCPLT based on limited data.[16] Pleomorphic liposarcoma typically shows a complex karyotype with numerous large-scale gains and losses, polyploidy, and occasional mutations in *TP53* and *NF1*, in contrast to the less disordered profile of ASCPLT.[17] However, it should be noted that 13q14 and *RB1* loss has been reported in a subset of pleomorphic liposarcomas, so the loss of *RB1*, especially out of context, does not allow distinction.[14]

DIAGNOSIS

Lipogenic neoplasm with infiltrating margins, variable amounts of atypical spindled or pleomorphic cells (sometimes multinucleated), and lipoblasts within a fibromyxoid stroma. Loss of Rb immunoexpression in a substantial subset of cases, correlating with *RB1* deletion, along with the absence of *MDM2* amplification, corroborates the diagnosis in challenging cases.[10]

PROGNOSIS

Although initial reports postulated ASCPLT as the malignant form of spindle cell/pleomorphic lipoma,[3–5] growing evidence suggests indolent clinical behavior with no documented evidence of progression, metastasis or mortality. However, a low but non-negligible risk for local recurrence was observed (approximately 10–15% of cases,

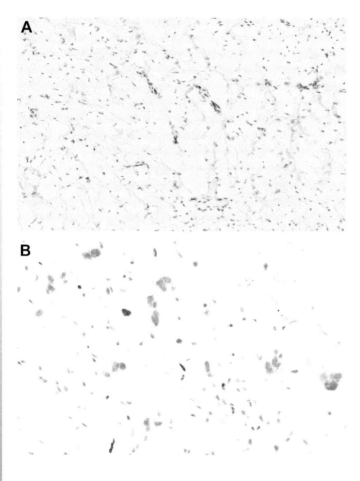

Fig. 5. Lost or deficient immunostaining for Rb is common in ASCPLT: (*A*). Atypical spindle cell lipomatous tumor at high magnification (400x original magnification), note the retained staining for Rb in endothelial cells and occasional smaller inflammatory cells. (*B*). Lost or deficient immunostaining for Rb is common in atypical pleomorphic lipomatous tumor, such as this example shown at high magnification (400x magnification): Retained staining is present in smaller, likely inflammatory cells and occasional spindle cells. Generally, staining in <10% of cells is regarded as evidence of Rb deficiency. (*From* Chen BJ, Mariño-Enríquez A, Fletcher CD, Hornick JL. Loss of retinoblastoma protein expression in spindle cell/pleomorphic lipomas and cytogenetically related tumors: an immunohistochemical study with diagnostic implications. Am J Surg Pathol. 2012 Aug;36(8):1119-28. https://doi.org/10.1097/PAS.0b013e31825d532d. PMID: 22790852.)

especially in patients with incomplete surgical excision) which warrants surgical excision with negative margins if feasible.[7,8,11] Recurrence of a previously diagnosed conventional spindle cell/pleomorphic lipoma warrants re-examination for the possibility of ASCPLT.

SUMMARY

ASCPLT is a newly described entity characterized by an ill-defined soft tissue tumor with a wide range of age and anatomical location, but a predilection for the limbs and limb girdles of adults. The tumors are composed of variable proportions of mature adipocytes, spindle cells, lipoblasts, and pleomorphic/multinucleated cells with mild to moderate atypia, within a fibromyxoid stroma. These tumors lack *MDM2* amplification but some can show the deletion of the *RB1* gene along with the nearest flanking genes. ASCPLT shows generally benign clinical behavior with low local recurrence risk and no metastatic risk (**Table 1**).

Fig. 6. Positive immunostaining for CD34 is frequently seen in ASCPLT (400x original magnification). (*A*). Atypical spindle cell lipomatous tumor at high magnification showing CD34 immunoreactivity. (*B*). CD34 positivity in atypical pleomorphic lipomatous tumor.

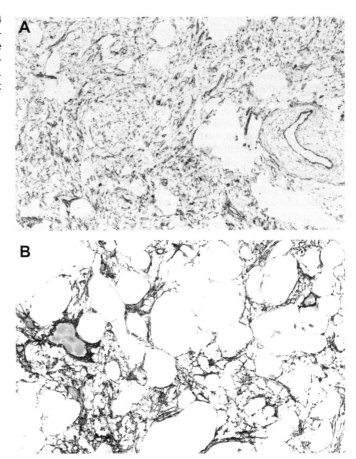

Table 1 Summary of ASCPLT features	
Epidemiology	Middle-aged adults (peak incidence 6th decade of life), M = F
Site	Limbs and limb girdles (subcutis > deep)
Gross	Ill-defined nodular mass, median size: 5–8.5 cm.
Morphology	Variably cellular lipogenic neoplasm with spindle to pleomorphic/multinucleated cells within a fibromyxoid stroma
Ancillary tests	IHC: Rb loss, CD34+/−, Molecular: *RB1* gene deletion
Prognosis	Low local recurrence rate (10–15%), No metastasis.
Differential diagnosis	SCL/PL, WDLPS/ALT, and PLPS

Abbreviations: F, female; IHC, immunohistochemistry; M, male; PLPS, pleomorphic liposarcoma; SCL/PL, Spindle cell/ pleomorphic lipoma; WDLPS/ALT, Well-differentiated liposarcoma/atypical lipomatous tumor.

CLINICS CARE POINTS

- The diagnosis of ASCPLT, and indeed lipogenic neoplasms as a group, is challenging due to the overlapping clinical and morphological features.

- Given this overlap, accurate diagnosis of ASCPLT requires careful correlation of clinical, imaging (eg, depth, margins), histopathologic, immunohistochemical (*RB1* loss), and molecular/genetic (eg, 13q14 deletion, absence of *MDM2* amplification) studies.

- Small biopsies or cytopathology preparations may not allow a definitive diagnosis beyond "lipogenic neoplasm" until molecular/genetic testing is completed.

- Despite initial concerns that ASCPLT represented the malignant counterpart of spindle cell lipoma, current evidence suggests that ASCPLT is benign with, at most, local recurrence potential.

DISCLOSURE

The authors have nothing to disclose.

REFERENCES

1. Fletcher CDM, Unni KK, Mertens F. Pathology and genetics of tumours of soft tissue and bone. WHO classification of tumours. 3rd edition. Lyon, France: IARC Press; 2002.
2. Fletcher CDM, Bridge JA, Hogendoorn P, et al. World health organization classification of tumours. pathology and genetics. Tumours of Soft Tissue and Bone. Lyon: IARC; 2013.
3. Dei Tos AP, Mentzel T, Newman PL, et al. Spindle cell liposarcoma, a hitherto unrecognized variant of liposarcoma. Analysis of six cases. Am J Surg Pathol 1994;18(9):913–21.
4. Mentzel T, Palmedo G, Kuhnen C. Well-differentiated spindle cell liposarcoma ('atypical spindle cell lipomatous tumor') does not belong to the spectrum of atypical lipomatous tumor but has a close relationship to spindle cell lipoma: clinicopathologic, immunohistochemical, and molecular analysis of six cases. Mod Pathol 2010;23(5):729–36.
5. Deyrup AT, Chibon F, Guillou L, et al. Fibrosarcoma-like lipomatous neoplasm: a reappraisal of so-called spindle cell liposarcoma defining a unique lipomatous tumor unrelated to other liposarcomas. Am J Surg Pathol 2013;37(9):1373–8.
6. Creytens D, van Gorp J, Savola S, et al. Atypical spindle cell lipoma: a clinicopathologic, immunohistochemical, and molecular study emphasizing its relationship to classical spindle cell lipoma. Virchows Arch 2014;465(1):97–108.
7. Mariño-Enriquez A, Nascimento AF, Ligon AH, et al. Atypical spindle cell lipomatous tumor: clinicopathologic characterization of 232 cases demonstrating a morphologic spectrum. Am J Surg Pathol 2017; 41(2):234–44.
8. Creytens D, Mentzel T, Ferdinande L, et al. "Atypical" pleomorphic lipomatous tumor: a clinicopathologic, immunohistochemical and molecular study of 21 cases, emphasizing its relationship to atypical spindle cell lipomatous tumor and suggesting a morphologic spectrum (atypical spindle cell/pleomorphic lipomatous tumor). Am J Surg Pathol 2017;41(11): 1443–55.
9. Bahadır B, Behzatoğlu K, Hacıhasanoğlu E, et al. Atypical spindle cell/pleomorphic lipomatous tumor: a clinicopathologic, immunohistochemical, and molecular study of 20 cases. Pathol Int 2018;68(10):550–6.
10. WHO Classification of Tumours Editorial Board. WHO Classification of tumours of soft tissue and bone. 5th ed. Lyon, France: IARC Press; 2020.
11. Evans HL. Anisometric cell lipoma: a predominantly subcutaneous fatty tumor with notable variation in fat cell size but not more than slight nuclear enlargement and atypia. AJSP Rev Rep 2016;21:195–9.
12. Michal M, Agaimy A, Contreras AL, et al. Dysplastic lipoma: a distinctive atypical lipomatous neoplasm with anisocytosis, focal nuclear atypia, p53 overexpression, and a lack of MDM2 gene amplification by FISH; a report of 66 cases demonstrating occasional multifocality and a rare association with retinoblastoma. Am J Surg Pathol 2018;42(11):1530–40.
13. Michal M, Agaimy A, Luiña Contreras A, et al. "Fat-rich" (spindle cell-poor) variants of atypical spindle cell lipomatous tumors show similar morphologic, immunohistochemical and molecular features as "dysplastic lipomas" are they related lesions? Am J Surg Pathol 2019;43(2):289–90.
14. Creytens D, Folpe AL, Koelsche C, et al. Myxoid pleomorphic liposarcoma-a clinicopathologic, immunohistochemical, molecular genetic and epigenetic study of 12 cases, suggesting a possible relationship with conventional pleomorphic liposarcoma. Mod Pathol 2021;34(11):2043–9.
15. Ohguri T, Hisaoka M, Kawauchi S, et al. Cytogenetic analysis of myxoid liposarcoma and myxofibrosarcoma by array-based comparative genomic hybridisation. J Clin Pathol 2006;59(9):978–83.
16. Suster S, Fisher C. Immunoreactivity for the human hematopoietic progenitor cell antigen (CD34) in lipomatous tumors. Am J Surg Pathol 1997;21(2):195–200.
17. Barretina J, Taylor BS, Banerji S, et al. Subtype-specific genomic alterations define new targets for soft-tissue sarcoma therapy. Nat Genet 2010;42(8): 715–21.

Soft Tissue Perivascular Epithelioid Cell Tumors

Phoebe M. Hammer, MD, Serena Y. Tan, MD*

KEYWORDS

• PEComa • Angiomyolipoma • TSC • TFE3

Key points

- PEComa family of tumors arising in soft tissue is rare and includes PEComas (not otherwise specified) and extrarenal angiomyolipomas.
- Most soft tissue PEComas are sporadic, with a small subset associated with tuberous sclerosis complex.
- PEComas are characterized by epithelioid and/or spindled cells with distinct perivascular orientation and variable myomelanocytic immunophenotype.
- Histologic criteria for malignancy include tumor size greater than 5 cm, increased mitoses, necrosis, infiltrative growth pattern, high nuclear grade, cellularity, and vascular invasion.
- PEComas show either *TSC1/2* loss or *TFE3*-rearrangements; molecular testing can be helpful diagnostically and therapeutically.

ABSTRACT

Perivascular epithelioid cell tumors (PEComas) are a heterogenous group of mesenchymal neoplasms with a mixed myomelanocytic immunophenotype. PEComa-family tumors include angiomyolipoma, lymphangioleiomyomatosis, and a large category of rare neoplasms throughout the body that are now classified under the umbrella term "PEComa." This review focuses on recent advances in the clinicopathological and molecular features of PEComas, with an emphasis on PEComas that originate in soft tissue.

OVERVIEW

Perivascular epithelioid cell tumors (PEComas) are a heterogenous family of mesenchymal neoplasms composed of morphologically distinct perivascular epithelioid cells (PECs) that usually express both melanocytic and smooth muscle markers.[1] In a correspondence published in 1991, Bonetti and colleagues[2] first proposed a link between HMB-45 immunoreactive clear cell "sugar" tumor (CCST) of the lung, the epithelioid component of angiomyolipomas (AMLs), and pulmonary lymphangioleiomyomatosis (LAM) and subsequently proposed the term "perivascular epithelioid cell" to describe the morphologically and immunohistochemically distinct cell found in these neoplasms.[3] They hypothesized that PECs might originate from the walls of blood vessels.[3] Zamboni and colleagues[4], in a report of pancreatic CCST, suggested the term *PEComa* to describe a neoplasm composed entirely of PECs. The PEComa family has since expanded to include rare visceral, intra-abdominal, soft tissue, bone, and cutaneous tumors described variously in the past as "primary

---

Department of Pathology, Stanford University School of Medicine, 1291 Welch Road, Lane Building L235, Stanford, CA 94305, USA
* Corresponding author. Department of Pathology, Stanford University School of Medicine, 1291 Welch Road, Lane Building L235, Stanford, CA 94305.
E-mail address: serenayt@stanford.edu

Surgical Pathology 17 (2024) 105–118
https://doi.org/10.1016/j.path.2023.06.002
1875-9181/24/© 2023 Elsevier Inc. All rights reserved.

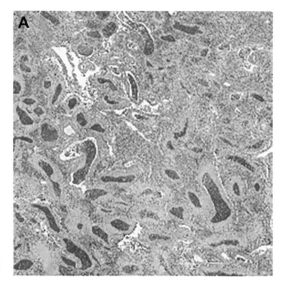

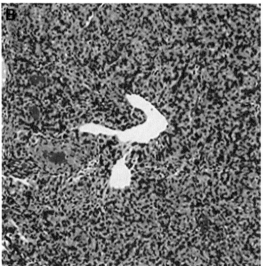

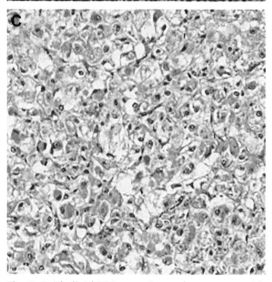

extrapulmonary sugar tumor,"[5] "abdominopelvic sarcoma of perivascular epithelioid cells,"[6] "clear cell myomelanocytic tumor of the falciform ligament/ligamentum teres,"[7] and "cutaneous clear cell myomelanocytic tumor,"[8] among others, and which are now broadly known as PEComas not otherwise specified or simply PEComas.[1] In the current WHO classification of soft tissue tumors, PEComas are subdivided into benign, intermediate, and malignant subgroups,[9] and related tumors include AML, epithelioid AML, and LAM.

This review describes the PEComa family tumors that arise in soft tissues, including PEComa, extrarenal AML, and extrarenal epithelioid AML (synonymous with PEComa).

CLINICAL FEATURES

PEComas have been reported in nearly all anatomic sites but are most frequently found in the genitourinary[10] and gynecologic tract,[11,12] followed by the gastrointestinal tract[13] and retroperitoneum,[14] and are rarely in somatic soft tissue, bone, and cutaneous sites.[1,8,15] A large variety of soft tissue sites have been described, including retroperitoneum, omentum and mesentery, abdominal wall, pelvic soft tissues, and deep and superficial soft tissue of the extremities and trunk.[1] There is an overall female predominance (approximately 5:1).[9]

Most PEComas show alterations in *TSC1* or *TSC2* including select subtypes, most notably renal AML and LAM, which show strong association with tuberous sclerosis complex (TSC), an autosomal dominant genetic disorder caused by germline mutations in either *TSC1* on chromosome 9 or *TSC2* on chromosome 16.[16] Among soft tissue PEComas, fibroma-like PEComas are highly associated with this syndrome.[17] Although most soft tissue PEComas are not associated with TSC,[1] many show alterations in *TSC2*. *TFE3* rearrangements represent an alternative molecular pathway of tumorigenesis. With rare exception,[18] *TFE3*-rearranged PEComas are not seen in patients with TSC,[19] tend to occur in young patients, and are usually seen in the gynecologic, genitourinary, and gastrointestinal tracts in addition to soft tissue sites.[13,20–22]

PATHOLOGIC FEATURES

PEComas are composed of epithelioid, spindled, and lipid-rich cells. Great variation is seen in the relative components,[23] with gross and

Fig. 1. Epithelioid PEComas. A vascular component is usually prominent and may include arteries/arterioles with hyalinized walls (*A*), hemangiopericytoma-like vessels (*B*), or delicate capillaries (*C*).

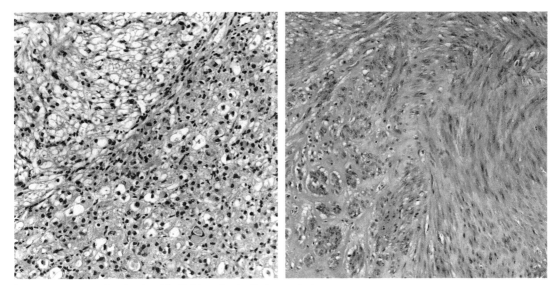

Fig. 2. PEComas with mixed epithelioid and spindled morphology.

microscopic features differing depending on predominant histomorphology. They are unencapsulated, may be well circumscribed or infiltrative,[1,13] and demonstrate a large size range. Microscopically, most soft tissue PEComas are lipid poor and demonstrate a mix of epithelioid and spindled cells, although predominant or pure epithelioid or spindled varieties exist. A lipomatous component is more prominent in classic AMLs, which tend to occur in the kidney but are found rarely in the soft tissue ("extrarenal AMLs"). *TFE3*-rearranged PEComas often demonstrate distinctive morphologic and immunophenotypic

features; other variations include sclerosing and fibroma-like PEComas and PECosis/ PEComatosis.

Many soft tissue PEComas have predominantly or purely epithelioid cells and are morphologically indistinguishable from renal epithelioid AMLs. In current practice, extrarenal epithelioid AMLs are referred to as "PEComas," even though the renal tumors continue to be referred to as epithelioid AMLs. The epithelioid cells are characteristically large and polygonal with clear to granular, eosinophilic cytoplasm, growing in sheet-like or nested arrangements,[1,13,14] and may be closely

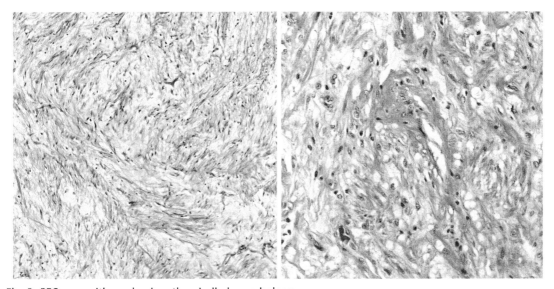

Fig. 3. PEComas with predominantly spindled morphology.

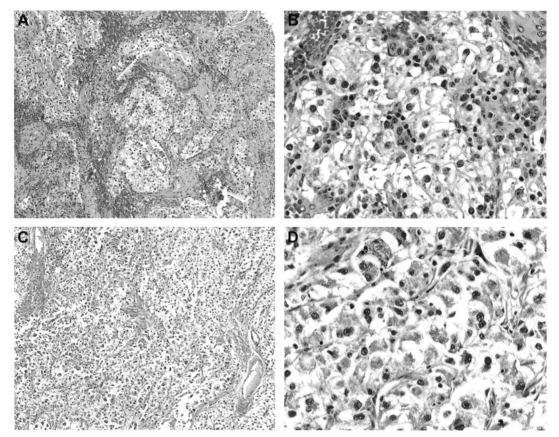

Fig. 4. Examples of *TFE3*-rearranged PEComas with nested and alveolar architecture. Tumors may have associated hemorrhage and inflammatory cells (*A, B*) and sometimes contain melanin pigment (*C, D*). (Photomicrographs courtesy of Andrew L Folpe, M.D., Rochester, Minnesota.).

associated with vessel walls, at times with a distinctive radial arrangement around the vascular lumens.[14,23] Their nuclei are round to ovoid with variably small nucleoli, although some tumors may show striking cytologic atypia with large, prominent nucleoli. A population of plump spindle cells may be present. There is nearly always a prominent vascular component, ranging from delicate, arborizing capillaries to thick hyalinized arterioles or arteries (**Fig. 1**).[1] Multinucleated giant cells, intranuclear pseudoinclusions, and melanin pigment are occasionally observed.[1,12,23]

Spindle cells in PEComas are typically myoid-appearing, with eosinophilic to clear cytoplasm and arranged in fascicles.[13] Although they usually accompany an epithelioid component (**Fig. 2**), pure or predominant spindle morphology has been described in a minority of PEComas[1,13] (**Fig. 3**), initially in a group of tumors called "clear cell myomelanocytic tumor" (CCMT), noted first in the falciform ligament/ligamentum teres and

subsequently in somatic soft tissue.[24] Since then, more examples of PEComas with pure spindle morphology have been reported.[1,13] We now recognize that CCMT is a morphologic variant of PEComas and not a distinct entity; hence, the use of this term is discouraged.[9]

TFE3-rearranged PEComas are usually epithelioid predominant and are characterized by nested or alveolar arrangement with associated delicate, thin-walled vasculature,[20] along with a variable spindle cell component[22,25] and collagenized stroma.[20] The epithelioid cells contain clear cytoplasm and demonstrate a range of atypia (**Fig. 4**).[22] Occasionally, they are morphologically indistinguishable from conventional PEComas.[25]

Sclerosing PEComas represent a subtype of PEComa that shows prominent stromal hyalinization (**Fig. 5**). They represent approximately 20% of PEComas, have a predilection for adult women and the retroperitoneum,[26] but have also been identified in the testis[27] and kidney,[28] rarely in

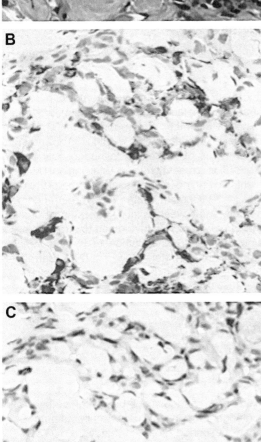

Fig. 5. Sclerosing PEComa (*A*) with stronger expression of desmin (*B*) than HMB45 (*C*).

the TSC context.[26,27] Morphologically, epithelioid cells are embedded in an abundant densely sclerotic stroma and lack the delicate vascular pattern typical of other PEComas.[26] Immunophenotypically, they show more muscle and less melanocytic marker expression than most PEComas (details in *Immunohistochemical Features*). In the absence of a frankly malignant component, sclerosing PEComas appear to behave in an indolent manner.[26]

Fibroma-like PEComa is a recently described subtype of PEComa that arises in association with TSC and resembles a fibroma by conventional morphology.[17] Fewer than 10 cases have been reported in the literature, most of which have been in younger patients and in soft tissue locations.[17,29–32] Grossly, tumors appear well-circumscribed, solid, and rubbery. Morphologically, they are characterized by bland spindled to stellate cells with no obvious organization embedded in abundant collagenous stroma. No cases have shown abnormalities in *TFE3*. All tested cases showed expression of at least one melanocytic and one muscle marker.[17,29–32] Given its apparent association with TSC, the identification of these morphologic features should raise consideration for germline testing if TSC is not already established.

While rare, extrarenal AMLs have been described in soft tissue sites, most commonly in the retroperitoneum.[33] In contrast to most other soft tissue PEComas, which are lipid poor and commonly epithelioid predominant, classic AMLs are characterized by "classic triphasic pattern" comprising a variable mix of mature adipose tissue, disorganized thick-walled blood vessels and spindled to epithelioid myoid cells (**Fig. 6**).[14] Owing to their atypical location, they present a unique diagnostic challenge.

PEComatosis/PECosis

PEComas usually appear as solitary tumors; however, rare reports of multifocal PEComas and/or microscopic proliferations of PECs have been described. The presence of multiple proliferations of PECs in a perivascular distribution has been termed "PEComatosis."[34] Less frequently, the term "PECosis" has been used to describe the phenomenon of multifocal PECs with distant dissemination through the capillary network,[35] leading to degeneration of surrounding tissue. PEComatosis has largely been described in the gynecologic tract and visceral locations, although it stands to reason that this phenomenon may occur in other anatomic sites.

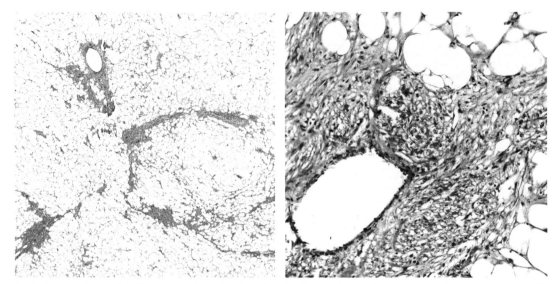

Fig. 6. Retroperitoneal AML composed predominantly of adipose tissue with interspersed vessels and a smaller smooth muscle component.

IMMUNOHISTOCHEMICAL FEATURES

PEComas are uniquely characterized by the expression of melanocytic and muscle markers, which show variable sensitivity (Table 1). HMB45 and cathepsin K are the most sensitive markers for PEComa in multiple anatomic sites.[1,12,36] Besides HMB45, other useful melanocytic markers include microphthalmia transcription factor (MiTF)[1,37] and MART-1/Melan-A.[1,11] More recently, PNL2 has shown moderate to high sensitivity[38,39] and may show more diffuse staining than HMB45.[38] Muscle markers are usually weaker, with focal or patchy expression.[1] Smooth muscle actin (SMA) is the most sensitive reported muscle marker[1,11,19,39–42]; desmin and caldesmon have shown a widely ranging sensitivity in studies on uterine PEComas.[1,19,39–41] Cytokeratin stains are negative.[1] S100 protein is generally negative, but may be at least weakly or focally positive in ~10% to 30% of tumors.[1,13] Although single-specific immunohistochemical stains for PEComas are lacking, the dual expression of at least one melanocytic marker and one muscle marker provides strong support for PEComa.

Variable relative expression of melanocytic and muscle markers has been observed in different subsets of PEComas, depending in part on their relative epithelioid and spindle components.[23] The epithelioid-appearing cells tend to express melanocytic markers more strongly than muscle markers, and myoid-appearing cells tend to show the opposite.[23] This variation has been described in greatest detail in the context of distinguishing uterine PEComas from smooth muscle and other mesenchymal lesions that can demonstrate myomelanocytic differentiation.[43,44] Sclerosing PEComas are reported to show the extensive expression of desmin, in contrast to other types of PEComas; although only patchy HMB45 is present, nuclear staining for MiTF is identified in most tumors and is usually extensive.[26] PEComas with *TFE3* rearrangement notably show weak or no expression of smooth muscle markers,[20,22] in addition to strong expression of HMB45 and cathepsin K, and variable expression of Melan-A.[20,22] *TFE3*-rearranged PEComas demonstrate strong expression of TFE3 by IHC, although a subset of *TFE3* fluorescence in situ hybridization (FISH)-negative tumors also show weak to moderate expression of TFE3.[20]

MOLECULAR FEATURES

Two major and distinct biological pathways of tumorigenesis in PEComa family tumors have been described—loss of function of *TSC1* or *TSC2* mutations and alternatively, *TFE3* gene rearrangements.[19] The loss of heterozygosity (LOH) of *TSC1* or *TSC2* is detected in PEComas arising in patients with TSC.[23,45] Outside of the TSC context, molecular studies in sporadic AMLs,[46,47] LAM,[48,49] and PEComas[19,50] have also demonstrated LOH in *TSC2*; *TSC1* LOH is only rarely detected in sporadic PEComas.[50] Pathogenic inactivating mutations of *TSC1/TSC2* lead to upregulation of the mammalian target of rapamycin (mTOR) pathway in PEComa family tumors that

Table 1
Immunohistochemical features of perivascular epithelioid cell tumors

Positive	Negative
Cathepsin K (100%)[1,13,30]	Cytokeratins (rare focal positivity)[1]
HMB45 (>90%)[1,13,30]	PAX8
MiTF (50–66%)[1,31]	S100 (focally positive in 10–30%)[1,14]
MART-1/Melan-A (46–72%)[1,31]	SOX1011
PNL2 (56%-85%)[32,33]	PRAME77
Smooth muscle actin (75–93%)[1,12,29,33–36]	CD34
Desmin (36–100%)[1,33–36]	DOG1
Caldesmon (64–92%)[1,33–36]	CD117 (focally positive in 30% of PEComas)[1]
Unique immunohistochemistry (IHC) Considerations	
Epithelioid predominant	Express melanocytic markers more strongly than myogenic markers
Spindled predominant	Express myogenic markers more strongly than melanocytic markers
TFE3-rearranged	Nuclear staining for TFE3[a], strong expression of melanocytic markers, weak or no expression of myogenic markers
Sclerosing subtype	Express myogenic markers (notably desmin) more extensively than melanocytic markers

[a] Note that TFE3 IHC is nonspecific and can be positive in tumors that lack TFE rearrangements.

can be targeted therapeutically with mTOR inhibitors.[51]

The second molecularly distinct subgroup of PEComas harbor TFE3 abnormalities[20] and involve approximately 20% of non-AML, non-LAM PEComas.[19] TFE3-rearranged PEComas demonstrate unique clinical and histopathologic characteristics that have already been described.

They lack the TSC2 LOH seen in the majority of PEComas, providing support for a biologically distinct pathogenesis,[52] and are important to recognize due in part to their differential response to mTOR inhibition. FISH for TFE3 rearrangements or detection of a TFE3 fusion via next-generation sequencing (NGS) can establish the molecular features. The lack of specificity of TFE3 IHC precludes diagnosis based on IHC alone, and molecular testing is needed to confirm TFE3 abnormalities.

Concurrent mutations in TP53 have also been identified in TSC-altered PEComas.[19,43,44] In malignant PEComas, up to 48% to 63% of tumors demonstrate TP53 abnormalities.[19,44,53] In addition, rare cases of both clinically benign and malignant PEComas in young adult patients with Li-Fraumeni syndrome (LFS) have been reported,[54,55] including concurrent diagnosis of PEComas in siblings with LFS.[54] The possible relationship between LFS and PEComas raises an important clinical consideration when diagnosing young patients with PEComa.

ASSESSMENT OF MALIGNANCY AND PROGNOSIS

PEComas show a range of clinical behavior, from benign to highly aggressive. Diagnostic criteria for aggressive behavior and malignancy continue to evolve.

The prognostic classification system established by Folpe and colleagues[1] divides PEComas into benign, uncertain malignant potential (UMP), and malignant based on six criteria: tumor size ≥ 5 cm, mitotic rate greater than 1/50 high-power fields, necrosis, an infiltrative growth pattern, high nuclear grade, and vascular invasion. Tumors lacking any of these features are considered benign, whereas tumors with at least two of these features are considered malignant (**Figs. 7** and **8**). The UMP category is applied to tumors with only a single histological feature, such as nuclear pleomorphism or multinucleated giant cells, or size ≥ 5 cm without other aggressive features.[1] These criteria have been substantiated for non-gynecologic sites.[56]

Molecular prognostic approaches for subsets of PEComas are starting to emerge. The prognostic understanding of TFE3-rearranged PEComas is incomplete, although cases with an aggressive clinical course and metastases have been reported. Multiple cases of malignant TFE3-rearranged or amplified PEComas have been recently reported,[18,21,57,58] with amplifications demonstrating a highly aggressive clinical course.

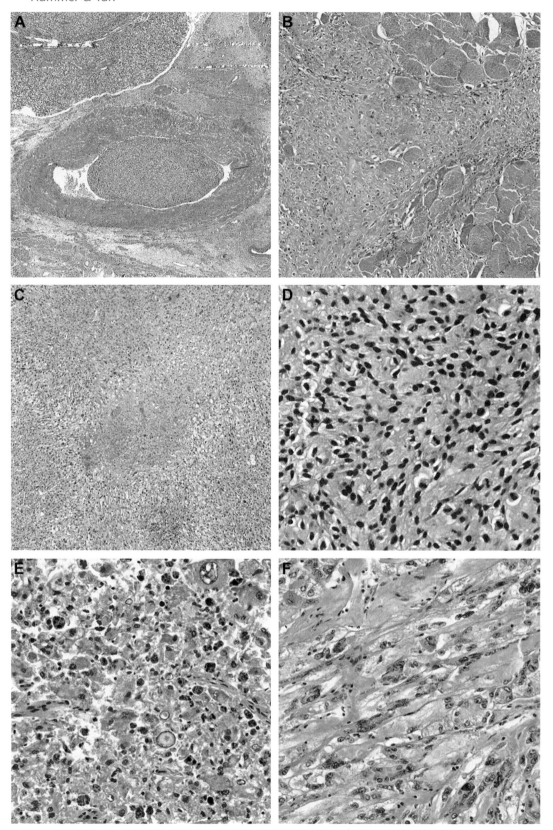

Fig. 7. Features of malignant PEComas. Malignant tumors may demonstrate vascular invasion (*A*), infiltration into surrounding tissue (*B*), necrosis (*C*), increased mitoses (*D*), and pleomorphic epithelioid (*E*) or spindled (*F*) cells.

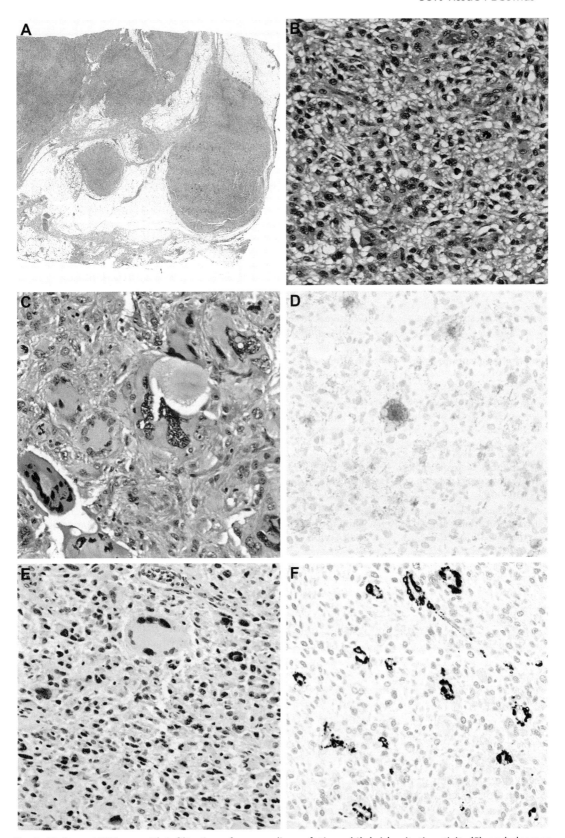

Fig. 8. Malignant PEComa with infiltration of surrounding soft tissue (*A*), brisk mitotic activity (*B*), and pleomorphic, multinucleated giant cells (*C*). The tumor is positive for HMB45 (*D*), negative for S100 protein (*E*), and shows patchy expression of smooth muscle actin (*F*).

Table 2
IHC and molecular characteristics of differential diagnostic considerations for epithelioid predominant perivascular epithelioid cell tumors

Diagnosis	IHC	Molecular Aberration
Metastatic carcinoma	Positive: cytokeratins (diffuse) Negative: melanocytic markers	
Metastatic melanoma	Positive: S100 (diffuse), Sox10 (diffuse) Negative: muscle markers	*BRAF* mutation
Clear cell sarcoma	Positive: S100 (diffuse), Sox10 (diffuse) Negative: muscle markers	*EWSR1-ATF1* or *EWSR-CREB1* fusions
Rhabdomyosarcoma	Positive: myogenin, myoD1, Pax7 Negative: melanocytic markers	*FOXO1* rearrangements in alveolar subtype
Epithelioid sarcoma/ malignant rhabdoid tumor	Positive: cytokeratins, EMA, CD34 Negative: INI1 (lost)	*hSNF5/INI1/SMARCB1* mutation testing
Epithelioid mesothelioma	Positive: cytokeratins, EMA, calretinin, WT1 Negative: melanocytic markers	
Lymphoma or plasma cell neoplasm	Positive: CD45 Negative: melanocytic and muscle markers	Variable[a]
Epithelioid angiosarcoma	Positive: CD31, ERG, CD34 Negative: melanocytic and muscle markers	
TFE3-rearranged neoplasms		
Alveolar soft part sarcoma	Negative: melanocytic markers	*ASPSCR1-TFE3* fusion
Metastatic Xp11.2 renal cell carcinoma	Positive: cytokeratins, PAX8 Negative: melanocytic markers, cathepsin K	Various *TFE3* and *TFEB* translocations
Metastatic melanotic Xp11 translocation renal cancers	Similar to *TFE3*-rearranged PEComas	Similar to *TFE3*-rearranged PEComas

[a] Targeted NGS panels are available for suspected hematolymphoid malignancies.

TP53 mutations may also portend malignancy in PEComas,[19,44,53] and PEComas in patients with LFS may behave aggressively.[54,55]

DIFFERENTIAL DIAGNOSIS

The differential diagnosis for PEComas is broad, and largely guided by the predominant histologic component and tumor location. An IHC panel is most useful and could be supplemented by molecular studies if necessary (**Tables 2–4**).

Given the expression of melanocytic markers, PEComas are frequently confused with metastatic melanoma or clear cell sarcoma[23] due in part to overlapping morphology, including epithelioid to spindled cells with prominent nucleoli and multinucleated cells and occasional pigmentation.[23]

These can usually be distinguished using IHC (see **Table 2**). Diffuse S100 expression is supportive of melanoma, which is generally negative or focal/weak in PEComas.[1] SOX10 is positive in the majority of melanoma and negative in PEComa.[10] If ambiguity remains, molecular studies may be helpful (see **Table 2**). PEComas with predominantly epithelioid morphology can also be confused with carcinomas, especially when located in visceral sites, rhabdomyosarcoma, epithelioid sarcoma, and epithelioid mesothelioma.

Spindle-predominant PEComas may be confused with smooth muscle neoplasms (see **Table 3**). In contrast to PEComas, smooth muscle neoplasms show diffusely eosinophilic cytoplasm, perinuclear vacuoles, and "cigar-shaped" nuclei.[23]

Table 3
IHC and molecular characteristics of differential diagnostic considerations for spindled predominant perivascular epithelioid cell tumors spindled predominant morphology

Diagnosis	IHC	Molecular Aberrations
Leiomyoma	Negative: melanocytic markers	
Leiomyosarcoma	Negative: Melan-A	
Gastrointestinal stromal tumor	Positive: DOG1 (diffuse), CD117 (diffuse), CD34, smooth muscle actin (focal) Negative: melanocytic markers, desmin	*KIT, PDGFRA* mutation testing

Leiomyosarcoma tends to have more cytologic atypia, frequent mitosis, and necrosis. Leiomyosarcomas may occasionally express HMB45[59] and cathepsin K; however, Melan-A is predictably negative.[10] Given inconsistencies in immunohistochemical profile, a panel of immunostains including HMB45, Melan-A, SMA, and desmin is recommended.[23] In the gastrointestinal tract, gastrointestinal stromal tumor (GIST) may enter the differential diagnosis. Because PEComas can rarely be positive for CD117,[1] GIST should be excluded with DOG1, a more specific stain. Finally, in the rare event of fat-predominant soft tissue PEComas (extrarenal AMLs), a variety of lipomatous tumors enter the differential and can be distinguished using a panel of IHC and molecular studies (see **Table 4**).

Given the occasional ambiguities in immunohistochemical staining patterns, molecular profiling has become increasingly important in distinguishing PEComas from other mesenchymal lesions with overlapping immunophenotypic profile,[60] with *TSC1* or *TSC2* alterations lending strong support for the diagnosis of PEComa in the appropriate morphologic context. When considering the diagnosis of PEComa, the detection of a *TFE3* rearrangement, while helpful, raises additional differential considerations of other *TFE3*-rearranged neoplasms, including Xp11.2 RCC, melanotic Xp11 translocation renal cancers, and alveolar soft part sarcoma (ASPS), which can also show alveolar or nested architecture, clear or eosinophilic cytology, immunoreactivity for TFE3, and *TFE3* rearrangements by FISH. Although metastatic Xp11.2-associated renal cancers are readily distinguished using IHC (see **Table 2**), melanotic Xp11 translocation renal cancers bear much greater similarity to PEComas in that they are usually positive for melanocytic markers and cathepsin K, whereas negative for PAX8 and muscle markers and most commonly involve an *SFPQ::TFE3* translocation[61]; hence, extrarenal soft tissue metastases of melanotic Xp11 translocation renal cancers may be virtually indistinguishable from soft tissue PEComas based on pathologic features alone. ASPS usually occurs in deep soft tissue sites of the extremities and more frequently shows vascular space invasion; unlike most *TFE3*-rearranged PEComas, ASPS is negative for HMB45 and Melan-A. Interestingly, ASPS harbors a unique

Table 4
IHC and molecular characteristics of differential diagnostic considerations for fat-predominant perivascular epithelioid cell tumors

Diagnosis	IHC	Molecular Aberrations
Lipoma	Negative: melanocytic markers	
Spindle cell lipoma	Positive: CD34 (diffuse) Negative: RB1 (loss) melanocytic markers, muscle markers	*RB1* mutation
Liposarcoma	Positive: MDM2 Negative: melanocytic markers	*MDM2, CDK4* amplifications

ASPSCR1::TFE3 translocation, which is strongly associated with ASPS and not typically found in PEComas, hence useful in their distinction.[22] However, the *ASPSCR1::TFE3* translocation was recently reported in three PEComa-like tumors expressing muscle markers,[62] suggesting that *TFE3*-rearranged neoplasms may lie on a continuum and our understanding of their distinctions is still evolving.

SUMMARY

PEComas arising in soft tissue are rare, constituting only a small subset of the complex PEComa family. Most present outside of the TSC context, but a minority appear to be associated with TSC. Although PEComas are unified by a distinctive perivascular growth, they have a diverse histologic spectrum with wide-ranging morphologic mimics. Their distinctive myomelanocytic immunophenotype has been a mainstay of PEComa diagnoses; however, molecular characterization, both of *TSC* alterations and *TFE3* rearrangements, is becoming a more common diagnostic tool in ambiguous cases. The increasingly widespread adoption of molecular sequencing, conversely, is challenging previously drawn boundaries between different diagnostic entities, especially among *TFE3*-rearranged neoplasms. Importantly, our understanding of the relationship between these dichotomous molecular pathways and how they may relate to the biology and prognosis of these tumors is still evolving.

DISCLOSURE

The authors have nothing to disclose.

CLINICS CARE POINTS

- PEComas are rare but increasingly recognized tumors with wide-ranging clinical behaviors that can be unpredictable.

- Distinguishing PEComas from melanocytic or smooth muscle neoplasms can be challenging and may involve a panel of immunohistochemical markers and possibly molecular studies.

- Evaluation for TFE3 rearrangements in PEComas can be important, particularly in aggressive cases, due to the potential of resistance to mTOR inhibition.

REFERENCES

1. Folpe AL, Mentzel T, Lehr HA, et al. Perivascular epithelioid cell neoplasms of soft tissue and gynecologic origin: a clinicopathologic study of 26 cases and review of the literature. Am J Surg Pathol 2005;29(12):1558–75.
2. Bonetti F, Pea M, Martignoni G, et al. Cellular heterogeneity in lymphangiomyomatosis of the lung. Hum Pathol 1991;22(7):727–8.
3. Bonetti F, Pea M, Martignoni G, et al. PEC and sugar. Am J Surg Pathol 1992;16(3):307–8.
4. Zamboni G, Pea M, Martignoni G, et al. Clear cell "sugar" tumor of the pancreas. A novel member of the family of lesions characterized by the presence of perivascular epithelioid cells. Am J Surg Pathol 1996;20(6):722–30.
5. Tazelaar HD, Batts KP, Srigley JR. Primary extrapulmonary sugar tumor (PEST): a report of four cases. Mod Pathol 2001;14(6):615–22.
6. Bonetti F, Martignoni G, Colato C, et al. Abdominopelvic sarcoma of perivascular epithelioid cells. Report of four cases in young women, one with tuberous sclerosis. Mod Pathol 2001;14(6):563–8.
7. Folpe AL, Goodman ZD, Ishak KG, et al. Clear cell myomelanocytic tumor of the falciform ligament/ligamentum teres: a novel member of the perivascular epithelioid clear cell family of tumors with a predilection for children and young adults. Am J Surg Pathol 2000;24(9):1239–46.
8. Mentzel T, Reisshauer S, Rütten A, et al. Cutaneous clear cell myomelanocytic tumour: a new member of the growing family of perivascular epithelioid cell tumours (PEComas). Clinicopathological and immunohistochemical analysis of seven cases. Histopathology 2005;46(5):498–504.
9. WHO Classification of Tumors Editorial Board. WHO classification of tumours of soft tissue and bone. 5th ed. Lyon, France: International Agency for Research on Cancer; 2020.
10. Hatfield BS, Mochel MC, Smith SC. Mesenchymal neoplasms of the genitourinary system: a selected review with recent advances in clinical, diagnostic, and molecular findings. Surg Pathol Clin 2018; 11(4):837–76.
11. Conlon N, Soslow RA, Murali R. Perivascular epithelioid tumours (PEComas) of the gynaecological tract. J Clin Pathol 2015;68(6):418–26.
12. Bennett JA, Braga AC, Pinto A, et al. Uterine PEComas: a morphologic, immunohistochemical, and molecular analysis of 32 tumors. Am J Surg Pathol 2018;42(10):1370–83.
13. Doyle LA, Hornick JL, Fletcher CD. PEComa of the gastrointestinal tract: clinicopathologic study of 35 cases with evaluation of prognostic parameters. Am J Surg Pathol 2013;37(12):1769–82.

14. Hornick JL, Fletcher CD. PEComa: what do we know so far? Histopathology 2006;48(1):75–82.

15. Auerbach A, Cassarino DS. Clear cell tumors of soft tissue. Surg Pathol Clin 2011;4(3):783–98.

16. Crino PB, Nathanson KL, Henske EP. The tuberous sclerosis complex. N Engl J Med 2006;355(13):1345–56.

17. Larque AB, Kradin RL, Chebib I, et al. Fibroma-like PEComa: a tuberous sclerosis complex-related lesion. Am J Surg Pathol 2018;42(4):500–5.

18. Schmiester M, Dolnik A, Kornak U, et al. TFE3 activation in a TSC1-altered malignant PEComa: challenging the dichotomy of the underlying pathogenic mechanisms. J Pathol Clin Res 2021;7(1):3–9.

19. Agaram NP, Sung YS, Zhang L, et al. Dichotomy of genetic abnormalities in PEComas with therapeutic implications. Am J Surg Pathol 2015;39(6):813–25.

20. Argani P, Aulmann S, Illei PB, et al. A distinctive subset of PEComas harbors TFE3 gene fusions. Am J Surg Pathol 2010;34(10):1395–406.

21. Lee W, HaDuong J, Sassoon A, et al. A liver transplant for local control in a pediatric patient with metastatic TFE3-associated perivascular epithelioid cell tumor (PEComa) to the liver. Case Rep Pathol 2021; 2021:3924565.

22. Schoolmeester JK, Dao LN, Sukov WR, et al. TFE3 translocation-associated perivascular epithelioid cell neoplasm (PEComa) of the gynecologic tract: morphology, immunophenotype, differential diagnosis. Am J Surg Pathol 2015;39(3):394–404.

23. Folpe AL, Kwiatkowski DJ. Perivascular epithelioid cell neoplasms: pathology and pathogenesis. Hum Pathol 2010;41(1):1–15.

24. Folpe AL, McKenney JK, Li Z, et al. Clear cell myomelanocytic tumor of the thigh: report of a unique case. Am J Surg Pathol 2002;26(6):809–12.

25. Maloney N, Giannikou K, Lefferts J, et al. Expanding the histomorphologic spectrum of TFE3-rearranged perivascular epithelioid cell tumors. Hum Pathol 2018;82:125–30.

26. Hornick JL, Fletcher CD. Sclerosing PEComa: clinicopathologic analysis of a distinctive variant with a predilection for the retroperitoneum. Am J Surg Pathol 2008;32(4):493–501.

27. Galea LA, Hildebrand MS, Boys A, et al. Sclerosing perivascular epithelioid cell tumour (PEComa) of the testis in a patient with tuberous sclerosis complex. Pathology 2023;55(1):143–6.

28. Zhao Y, Bui MM, Spiess PE, et al. Sclerosing PEComa of the kidney: clinicopathologic analysis of 2 cases and review of the literature. Clin Genitourin Cancer 2014;12(5):e229–32.

29. Bajaj G, Lindberg MR, Chee W, et al. Fibroma-like PEComa: a newly recognized soft tissue neoplasm in tuberous sclerosis patients-imaging features and review of literature. Skeletal Radiol 2022;51(4): 881–7.

30. Harvey JP, Suster DI, Raskin KA, et al. Intra-articular fibroma-like perivascular epithelioid tumor (PEComa) mimicking tenosynovial giant cell tumor, diffuse type. Skeletal Radiol 2019;48(6):965–9.

31. Odoño EIG, Tan KB, Tay SY, et al. Cutaneous "fibroma-like" perivascular epithelioid cell tumor: a case report and review of literature. J Cutan Pathol 2020;47(6):548–53.

32. Ramezanpour S, Horvai AE, Zimel M, et al. Fibroma-like perivascular epithelioid cell tumor: a rare case in a long bone. Skeletal Radiol 2021;50(4):821–5.

33. Minja EJ, Pellerin M, Saviano N, et al. Retroperitoneal extrarenal angiomyolipomas: an evidence-based approach to a rare clinical entity. Case Rep Nephrol 2012;2012:374107.

34. Fadare O, Parkash V, Yilmaz Y, et al. Perivascular epithelioid cell tumor (PEComa) of the uterine cervix associated with intraabdominal "PEComatosis": a clinicopathological study with comparative genomic hybridization analysis. World J Surg Oncol 2004;2: 35.

35. Weinreb I, Howarth D, Latta E, et al. Perivascular epithelioid cell neoplasms (PEComas): four malignant cases expanding the histopathological spectrum and a description of a unique finding. Virchows Arch 2007;450(4):463–70.

36. Martignoni G, Bonetti F, Chilosi M, et al. Cathepsin K expression in the spectrum of perivascular epithelioid cell (PEC) lesions of the kidney. Mod Pathol 2012;25(1):100–11.

37. Acosta AM, Adley BP. Predicting the behavior of perivascular epithelioid cell tumors of the uterine corpus. Arch Pathol Lab Med 2017;141(3):463–9.

38. Gulavita P, Fletcher CDM, Hirsch MS. PNL2: an adjunctive biomarker for renal angiomyolipomas and perivascular epithelioid cell tumours. Histopathology 2018;72(3):441–8.

39. Valencia-Guerrero A, Pinto A, Anderson WJ, et al. PNL2: a useful adjunct biomarker to HMB45 in the diagnosis of uterine perivascular epithelioid cell tumor (PEComa). Int J Gynecol Pathol 2020;39(6): 529–36.

40. Bennett JA, Oliva E. Perivascular epithelioid cell tumors (PEComa) of the gynecologic tract. Genes Chromosomes Cancer 2021;60(3):168–79.

41. Vang R, Kempson RL. Perivascular epithelioid cell tumor ('PEComa') of the uterus: a subset of HMB-45-positive epithelioid mesenchymal neoplasms with an uncertain relationship to pure smooth muscle tumors. Am J Surg Pathol 2002;26(1):1–13.

42. Schoolmeester JK, Howitt BE, Hirsch MS, et al. Perivascular epithelioid cell neoplasm (PEComa) of the gynecologic tract: clinicopathologic and immunohistochemical characterization of 16 cases. Am J Surg Pathol 2014;38(2):176–88.

43. Bennett JA, Ordulu Z, Pinto A, et al. Uterine PEComas: correlation between melanocytic marker

expression and TSC alterations/TFE3 fusions. Mod Pathol 2022;35(4):515–23.

44. Anderson WJ, Dong F, Fletcher CDM, et al. A clinicopathologic and molecular characterization of uterine sarcomas classified as malignant PEComa. Am J Surg Pathol 2023. https://doi.org/10.1097/PAS.0000000000002028.

45. Henske EP, Scheithauer BW, Short MP, et al. Allelic loss is frequent in tuberous sclerosis kidney lesions but rare in brain lesions. Am J Hum Genet 1996;59(2):400–6.

46. Henske EP, Neumann HP, Scheithauer BW, et al. Loss of heterozygosity in the tuberous sclerosis (TSC2) region of chromosome band 16p13 occurs in sporadic as well as TSC-associated renal angiomyolipomas. Genes Chromosomes Cancer 1995;13(4):295–8.

47. Qin W, Bajaj V, Malinowska I, et al. Angiomyolipoma have common mutations in TSC2 but no other common genetic events. PLoS One 2011;6(9):e24919.

48. Smolarek TA, Wessner LL, McCormack FX, et al. Evidence that lymphangiomyomatosis is caused by TSC2 mutations: chromosome 16p13 loss of heterozygosity in angiomyolipomas and lymph nodes from women with lymphangiomyomatosis. Am J Hum Genet 1998;62(4):810–5.

49. Carsillo T, Astrinidis A, Henske EP. Mutations in the tuberous sclerosis complex gene TSC2 are a cause of sporadic pulmonary lymphangioleiomyomatosis. Proc Natl Acad Sci U S A 2000;97(11):6085–90.

50. Pan CC, Jong YJ, Chai CY, et al. Comparative genomic hybridization study of perivascular epithelioid cell tumor: molecular genetic evidence of perivascular epithelioid cell tumor as a distinctive neoplasm. Hum Pathol 2006;37(5):606–12.

51. Dickson MA, Schwartz GK, Antonescu CR, et al. Extrarenal perivascular epithelioid cell tumors (PEComas) respond to mTOR inhibition: clinical and molecular correlates. Int J Cancer 2013;132(7):1711–7.

52. Malinowska I, Kwiatkowski DJ, Weiss S, et al. Perivascular epithelioid cell tumors (PEComas) harboring TFE3 gene rearrangements lack the TSC2 alterations characteristic of conventional PEComas: further evidence for a biological distinction. Am J Surg Pathol 2012;36(5):783–4.

53. Wagner AJ, Ravi V, Riedel RF, et al. -Sirolimus for patients with malignant perivascular epithelioid cell tumors. J Clin Oncol 2021;39(33):3660–70.

54. Galera López MDM, Márquez Rodas I, Agra Pujol C, et al. Simultaneous diagnosis of liver PEComa in a family with known Li-Fraumeni syndrome: a case report. Clin Sarcoma Res 2020;10(1):24.

55. Neofytou K, Famularo S, Khan AZ. PEComa in a young patient with known li-fraumeni syndrome. Case Rep Med 2015;2015:906981.

56. Bleeker JS, Quevedo JF, Folpe AL. "Malignant" perivascular epithelioid cell neoplasm: risk stratification and treatment strategies. Sarcoma 2012;2012:541626.

57. Zhang Y, Wei X, Teng X, et al. p53 aberration and TFE3 gene amplification may be predictors of adverse prognosis in epithelioid angiomyolipoma of the kidney. Diagn Pathol 2023;18(1):14.

58. Argani P, Zhang L, Sung YS, et al. A novel RBMX-TFE3 gene fusion in a highly aggressive pediatric renal perivascular epithelioid cell tumor. Genes Chromosomes Cancer 2020;59(1):58–63.

59. Simpson KW, Albores-Saavedra J. HMB-45 reactivity in conventional uterine leiomyosarcomas. Am J Surg Pathol 2007;31(1):95–8.

60. Selenica P, Conlon N, Gonzalez C, et al. Genomic profiling aids classification of diagnostically challenging uterine mesenchymal tumors with myomelanocytic differentiation. Am J Surg Pathol 2021;45(1):77–92.

61. Argani P, Zhong M, Reuter VE, et al. TFE3-Fusion variant analysis defines specific clinicopathologic associations among Xp11 translocation cancers. Am J Surg Pathol 2016;40(6):723–37.

62. Argani P, Wobker SE, Gross JM, et al. PEComa-like neoplasms characterized by ASPSCR1-TFE3 fusion: another face of TFE3-related mesenchymal neoplasia. Am J Surg Pathol 2022;46(8):1153–9.

Sclerosing Epithelioid Fibrosarcoma

Laura M. Warmke, MD[a], Wendong Yu, MD, PhD[b], Jeanne M. Meis, MD[b],*

KEYWORDS

- Sclerosing epithelioid fibrosarcoma • Low-grade fibromyxoid sarcoma • MUC4 • EWSR1 • FUS
- CREB3L1 • CREB3L2 • KMT2A

Key points

- SEF is under-recognized in biopsies due to bland fibrous areas and bland cytologic features
- A small cell malignancy with sclerosis or osteoid-like foci should alert the pathologist to consider SEF
- Classification as SEF depends upon the integration of clinical and histological findings and extended sarcoma fusion testing in most instances
- SEF with *YAP1::KMT2A* fusion may represent a distinct entity or heterogeneous group of tumors
- The histologic differential diagnosis of SEF is wide and includes low-grade fibromyxoid sarcoma, malignant myoepithelioma, and ossifying fibromyxoid tumor of soft parts as the primary considerations
- SEF is a high-grade sarcoma, recalcitrant to chemotherapy

ABSTRACT

Sclerosing epithelioid fibrosarcoma (SEF) is a distinctive sarcoma that may arise in nearly any soft tissue site or bone. While there has been past controversy as to whether it is related to low-grade fibromyxoid sarcoma (LGFMS), it has been shown to behave far more aggressively than LGFMS. SEF has a propensity to metastasize to the lungs and bone and arise within the abdominal cavity. Histologically, it is characterized by uniform nuclei embedded in a densely collagenous stroma simulating osteoid. By immunohistochemistry, it is often strongly positive for MUC4. The majority (75%) have EWSR1 gene rearrangement, most commonly with CREB3L1 as a fusion partner, although a variety of FUS/EWSR1 and CREB3L1/CREB3L2/CREB3L3 fusions have been described in addition to others. SEF is currently recalcitrant to nearly all chemotherapy and radiation therapy.

HISTORICAL OVERVIEW OF SCLEROSING EPITHELIOID FIBROSARCOMA

Sclerosing epithelioid fibrosarcoma (SEF) was originally documented 30 years ago[1] and fully described as a unique entity in 1995.[2] The salient clinicopathologic features of SEF were those of a deep-seated mass that histologically comprised small, deceptively bland, angulated, uniform cells arranged in nests and cords that were embedded in a fibrotic or hyalinized matrix. The presence of clear cell zones surrounding nuclei, resulting in a lacunar-like appearance, was also a prominent feature.[1,2] Minor areas of conventional, low-grade fibrosarcoma were observed in several cases. Occasional foci reminiscent of low-grade fibromyxoid sarcoma (LGFMS) or low-grade myxofibrosarcoma were noted in the original publication,[3,4] as were fibroma-like zones, cyst formation, and calcification. Ultrastructural studies confirmed the histological impression of fibroblastic differentiation,[5,6] hence the lesion was

---

The authors have no disclosures.
^a Department of Pathology and Laboratory Medicine, Indiana University, IU Health Pathology Laboratory, 350 W 11th Street, Room 4086, Indianapolis, IN 46202, USA; ^b Department of Pathology and Laboratory Medicine, The University of Texas MD Anderson Cancer Center, 1515 Holcombe Boulevard, Pathology Unit #085, Houston, TX 77030, USA
* Corresponding author. Department of Pathology and Laboratory Medicine, The University of Texas MD Anderson Cancer Center, Un #085, 1515 Holcombe Boulevard, Houston, TX 77005.
E-mail address: JMMeis@mdanderson.org

Surgical Pathology 17 (2024) 119–139
https://doi.org/10.1016/j.path.2023.06.009
1875-9181/24/© 2023 Elsevier Inc. All rights reserved.

called fibrosarcoma, despite the dwindling popularity of that diagnosis. Most patients had a protracted clinical course, even with lung metastases; therefore, this lesion was originally viewed as a low-grade sarcoma although there was no question as to its malignancy.[1,2]

Subsequent series confirmed the distinctness of SEF as an entity and its fibroblastic nature, although the clinical behavior was shown to be somewhat more aggressive than initially described.[7–10] The relative rarity of SEF compared to LGFMS, unfamiliarity with its prototypical histology, and the occurrence of fibrotic forms of LGFMS resulted in several reports emphasizing histologic overlap between the 2 lesions and led some investigators to postulate a close relationship between LFGMS and SEF.[8,11–13] Subsequent detection of FUS::CREB3L2 in the overwhelming majority of LGFMS (including those with fibrosing or so-called hybrid areas) was construed as further supporting a relationship between the 2.[14–16] Immunohistochemical detection of strong MUC4 positivity in both LGFMS and SEF provided additional impetus for considering these 2 tumors as part of a morphologic spectrum.[17,18]

However, a genetic profile of SEF gradually began to emerge in which FUS was rarely detected in classical or "pure" cases of SEF.[19] Subsequent molecular studies showed EWSR1::-CREB3L1 to be the predominant fusion in this lesion.[20,21] These findings led to the documentation of primary SEF in a variety of viscera and organs as well as skeletal sites which had been previously misdiagnosed as osteosarcoma.[22–33]

Molecular variants and subsets of SEF, or even wholly different tumors that simulate SEF, continue to emerge with in-depth molecular analysis.[34–36] Most importantly, however, the biologic behavior of SEF has been found to be significantly more aggressive than LGFMS, and it also behaves as a higher-grade sarcoma than originally believed.[9] Moreover, it has proven to be recalcitrant to typical sarcoma regimens as well as experimental modalities at this juncture.[37,38] As such, its distinction from LGFMS is important for appropriate patient treatment and development of more effective treatment modalities.

MORPHOLOGIC AND IMMUNOHISTOCHEMICAL FEATURES OF SCLEROSING EPITHELIOID FIBROSARCOMA

HISTOLOGIC FEATURES OF SCLEROSING EPITHELIOID FIBROSARCOMA

SEF is typically deep-seated, involving fascia, skeletal muscle, periosteum, and bone.[1,2,8,30,33] Its margins are usually circumscribed although infiltrative areas may be seen. The majority of SEF are hyalinized, with deeply acidophilic rope-like strands of collagen or a homogeneous hyalinized matrix that often resembles osteoid; this in turn surrounds strands, cords, nests, or pseudo-acinar groups of small cells. The cells are uniform and have scant cytoplasm that is usually clear but occasionally eosinophilic. The appearance of clear cytoplasm is often attributed to retraction artefact due to extensive hyalinization, resulting in a resemblance to lacunae. However, histochemical and ultrastructural studies confirm the presence of scant amounts of cytoplasmic glycogen. Nuclei are usually round to oval, with finely and evenly dispersed chromatin, although occasionally the chromatin is coarser and hyperchromatic. Nucleoli are small and inconspicuous.[1,2,8,9]

A less common appearance of SEF is that of a highly cellular small-cell sarcoma with scant acidophilic cytoplasm. Cells are uniform with a high N:C ratio. Closer inspection reveals a delicate osteoid-like or filigree pattern of collagen deposition, which is the best clue that one is dealing with SEF.[9,39]

Focal areas of low-grade conventional fibrosarcoma may be seen, as well as minor hypocellular myxoid zones that overlap with low-grade fibromyxoid sarcoma, low-grade myxofibrosarcoma, and even desmoid. Other non-specific patterns are foci that resemble cellular fibrous histiocytoma, fibroma-like areas, cyst formation, and focal cartilaginous and osseous metaplasia. The overall impression of a lesion as highly sclerotic, regardless of the presence of these minor features, is the best guide to distinguish SEF from LGFMS and will avoid confusion with LGFMS or so-called hybrid forms.[2,8,40]

ULTRASTRUCTURE OF SCLEROSING EPITHELIOID FIBROSARCOMA

Ultrastructurally, SEF displays features of fibroblasts, despite rare, focal weak immunohistochemical positivity for EMA, S100 protein, or keratin. The constituent cells are devoid of external lamina although they are surrounded by dense bundles or whorls of collagen which may have calcifications and thereby simulate osteoid. Individual cells contain whorls of intermediate filaments that correspond immunohistochemically to vimentin. There is abundant rough endoplasmic reticulum that is often distended with granular to fibrillar material and intracytoplasmic collagen may occasionally be seen.[2,6,8]

IMMUNOHISTOCHEMISTRY OF SCLEROSING EPITHELIOID FIBROSARCOMA

Immunohistochemistry for MUC4, a high molecular weight transmembrane glycoprotein, can be an especially useful adjunct in the diagnosis of SEF, as well as LGFMS, as it is expressed strongly and diffusely in practically all LGFMS and most SEF.[17,18] One must remember it will not distinguish between LGFMS or SEF, which is primarily a morphologic distinction as mentioned above. Moreover, MUC4 is not entirely restricted to these 2 sarcomas, as it may be seen in alveolar rhabdomyosarcoma,[41] and more importantly, ossifying fibromyxoid tumor of soft parts[42] and myoepithelial carcinomas.[18] The latter 2 entities may closely simulate SEF, particularly in core biopsies which are the most common method of tissue procurement; thus, an expanded immunohistochemical panel and molecular studies, as well as close imaging correlation, are usually necessary to distinguish between these lesions on limited material.

CYTOLOGY OF SCLEROSING EPITHELIOID FIBROSARCOMA

As there is little written in the literature regarding fine needle aspirations (FNA) of SEF,[43–45] we reviewed 9 samples (3 primary and 6 metastatic sites) from 6 patients diagnosed with SEF from our institution within the last 10 years. The diagnoses were supported by the identification of at least one of the following: classical gene fusion for SEF, EWSR1 gene rearrangement, or positive MUC4 immunostaining.

The cytologic features seen in SEF mirror those seen by histologic examination although cellular preservation is better in some aspirates due to severe crush artifact in core biopsies. As expected, the most fibrotic variants yield paucicellular samples, whereas the hypercellular variants have good cell yields. The less cellular yields with sclerotic fibrous tissue have better preservation of tumor cell morphology at the periphery of the tissue fragments. Most of the tumor cells are either singly arranged or in small clusters, often in a background of granular debris. Tumor cells typically have a minimal to moderate amount of eccentrically located cytoplasm. Nuclei are round, oval, or short and spindled in shape with mild pleomorphism. Chromatin is typically fine with occasional small nucleoli; a few have irregularly distributed chromocenters. The nuclear membrane is typically smooth with slight irregularity; however, a few cases demonstrate more pronounced pleomorphism with markedly irregular nuclear membranes. Occasional nuclear inclusions and rare mitotic figures are also seen.

The salient histologic and cytologic features of SEF in comparison to LGFMS with relevant immunohistochemistry and ultrastructure are summarized in **Table 1**. See also **Figs. 1–5** of SEF, which is more stereotypical in comparison to

Table 1
SEF and LGFMS: comparison of typical histologic, cytologic, immunohistochemical and ultrastructural features

	SEF	LGFMS
Architecture	Nests, pseudo alveoli, cords, single files; occasional fascicles	Whorls, swirls, and vague fascicles; tigroid pattern
Matrix	Fibrous, ropey, sclerotic, osteoid-like; occasional metaplastic bone and cartilage	Myxoid to fibrous; chondro-osseous metaplasia rare; highly vascular with perivascular cells
Cell shape and density	Uniform and cellular; round to ovoid in shape, occasionally spindled	Spindled and occasionally epithelioid; relatively hypocellular
Cytoplasm	Clear and occasionally eosinophilic; well demarcated	Eosinophilic and syncytial
Nuclear shape	Rounded or ovoid; occasionally spindled; usually smooth membrane contours, occasionally irregular	Ovoid; occasionally epithelioid; minimal pleomorphism
Chromatin	Finely dispersed with small nucleoli; occasionally hyperchromatic	Finely dispersed; occasionally hyperchromatic
Mitotic activity	Variable, usually less than 10/10 hpf	Absent to sparse
Necrosis	Occasionally present	Typically absent
Immunohistochemistry	MUC4 positive in ~80%; EMA positive (focal)	MUC4 positive in ~100%; EMA positive (weak)
Ultrastructure	Fibroblastic features with abundant RER, extra-cellular collagen; osteoid-like collagen	Prominent myxoid stroma with rare hyalinized zones

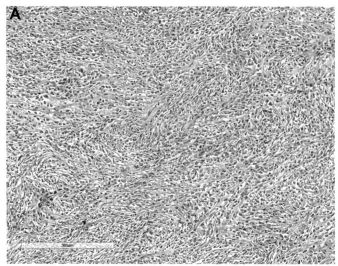

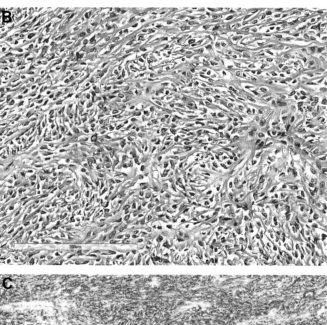

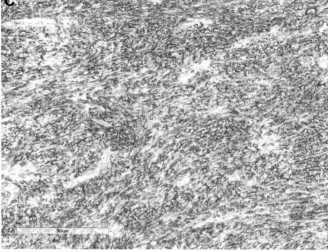

Fig. 1. (*A–C*). Sclerosing epithelioid fibrosarcoma removed from the back of a 53-year-old man, clinically believed to be a lipoma. (*A* and *B*) Classical histology of SEF with uniform and angulated cells and ropey collagen strands. (*C*) Diffuse immunohistochemical staining for MUC4.

Fig. 2. (*A–C*). Another typical SEF which involved the parotid gland in an elderly woman with a recurrence that revealed an *EWSR1::CREB3L3* fusion. (*A*) Salivary gland at left, infiltrated by tumor. (*B*) Regular cord-like and pseudo-alveolar arrangements of cells in a fibrous matrix. (*C*) FNA, Pap stain of local recurrence showing bland nuclei with slightly irregular nuclear contours and background fibrous matrix.

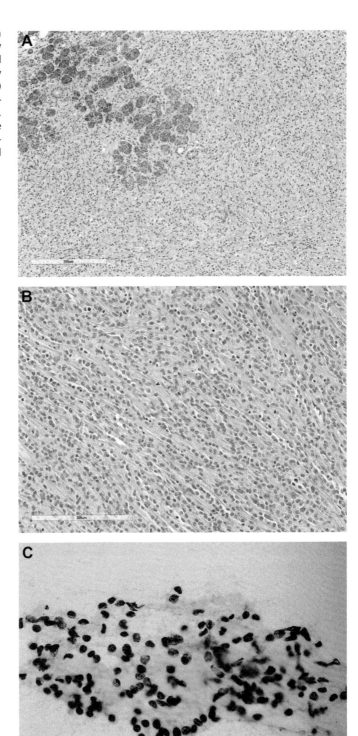

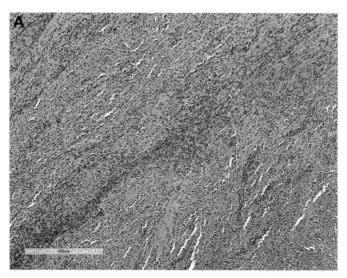

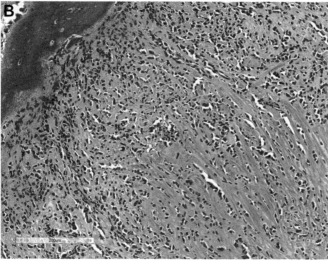

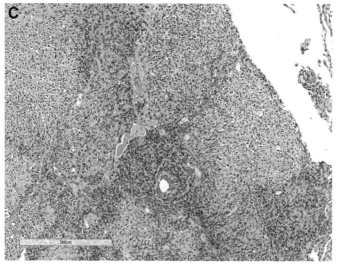

Fig. 3. (*A–C*). Densely cellular example of SEF arising in the iliacus of a 53-year-old woman with a *CHEK2* germline mutation. (*A* and *B*) The primary tumor has areas of dense sclerosis simulating osteoid, and bone formation (upper left) was also seen (*B*). The patient developed lung metastasis, which was highly cellular and simulated osteosarcoma (*C*), and bone metastasis. The tumor demonstrated *EWSR1::CREB3L1* fusion and was MUC4-positive.

Fig. 4. (*A–H*). SEF of abdominal cavity. (*A*) Large abdominal mass with colon perforation (air pocket, left abdomen) and multiple liver metastases. (*B*) Initial core biopsy of liver reveals severe crush artifact of tumor cells with preservation of thick collagen bands that raised suspicion of SEF. (*C* and *D*) Diffuse and strong MUC4 positivity in the liver biopsy with negative hepatocytes (*C*, right) and prominent staining in crushed cytoplasm

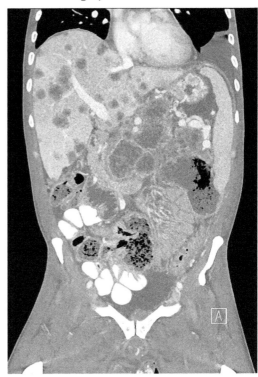

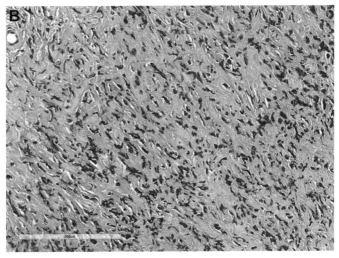

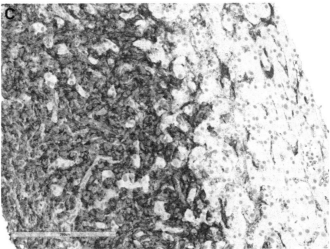

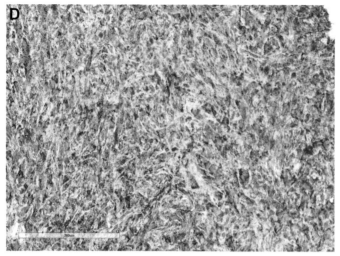

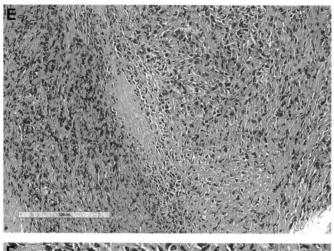

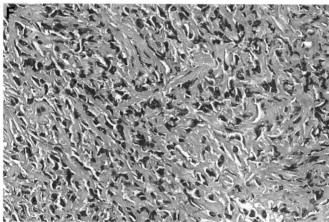

Fig. 4. and *D*) Diffuse and strong MUC4 positivity in the liver biopsy with negative hepatocytes (*C*, right) and prominent staining in crushed cytoplasm (*D*). Subsequent metastases to soft tissue in neck (*E* and *F*) again show the thick bands of collagen with poorly preserved and slightly pleomorphic nuclear features. Cytological preparation of intact tumor cells of neck metastases on Pap stain

LGFMS (**Figs. 6** and **7**) that can illustrate a potentially wide spectrum.

MOLECULAR FEATURES OF SCLEROSING EPITHELIOID FIBROSARCOMA

The most common gene rearrangement in SEF is *EWSR1::CREB3L1*, with fewer cases showing *EWSR1::CREB3L2* fusion.[9,16,20,21] In contrast, *FUS::CREB3L2* is the most common gene rearrangement identified in LGFMS, with a small subset showing *FUS::CREB3L1*.[14,15] Not surprisingly, there are rare LGFMS with *EWSR1::CREB3L1* translocations,[46] while some cases of so-called pure SEF (without recognizable LGFMS-like areas) have demonstrated *FUS::CREB3L2* fusions[16] or

Fig. 4. (*G*) and Diff-Quik stain (*H*) revealing eccentric nuclei and irregular nuclear features. The primary tumor showed *FUS::KIAA1549* and *KIAA1549::-CREB3L2* fusions. The patient expired 5 months later.

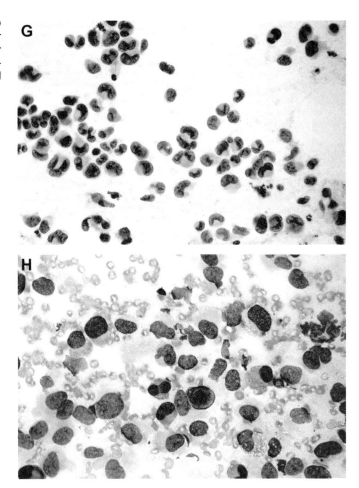

FUS rearrangement by fluorescence in situ hybridization (FISH).[19] Those cases with so-called hybrid features of SEF and LGFMS have shown primarily *FUS::CREB3L2* fusions, raising the possibility that these may be sclerosing variants of LGFMS.[47]

In addition to the various combinations of *EWSR1/FUS* with *CREB3L1/CREB3L2*, *FUS::CREM*, *PAX5::-CREB3L1*, *EWSR1::CREB3L3*, and *HEY1::NCOA2* fusions have been reported in SEF.[47–49] A possible subset of SEF that is negative for MUC4 with *YAP1::KMT2A* gene fusions has been reported by a few investigators in addition to a case of *PRRX1::KMT2D* gene fusion (see later in discussion).[34,35]

The cumulative experience with SEF molecular analysis of 22 cases seen at our institution is similar with the literature; 14 (64%) showed *EWSR1::CREB3L1* fusions, 3 (14%) *YAP1::KMT2A*, 2 (9%) *EWSR1::CREB3L2*, one *EWSR1::CREB3L3*, one *FUS::CREB3L2*, and one case with 2 fusions including *FUS::KIAA1549* and *KIAA1549::CREB3L2*.

MUC4-NEGATIVE SCLEROSING EPITHELIOID FIBROSARCOMA AND *KMT2A*-REARRANGED SARCOMA

A new and distinct subset of fibroblastic tumors characterized by *KMT2A* gene rearrangements and SEF-like morphology has been described.[50] Gene rearrangements involving *KMT2A* (lysine methyltransferase 2A), formerly known as *MLL1* (mixed-lineage leukemia), have been reported in several neoplasms, including a small subset of acute leukemias with poor prognosis,[51] thymoma,[52] and neuroblastoma.[53] In the realm of sarcomas, *KMT2A* is frequently fused to *YAP1* (Yes-associated protein 1), resulting in tumors with distinct SEF-like features, composed of epithelioid and spindle cells arranged in cords in a densely sclerotic stroma. In 2018, Watson and colleagues[54] reported the first case of a "sclerosing fibrosarcoma" with *YAP1::KMT2A* fusion involving the chest wall of a 35-year-old female. Since then,

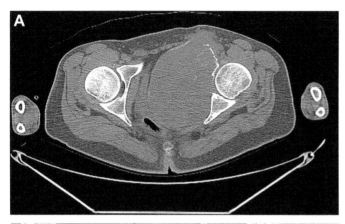

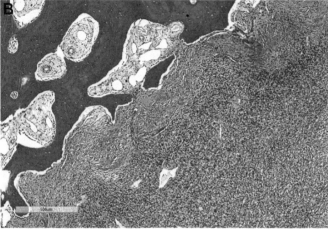

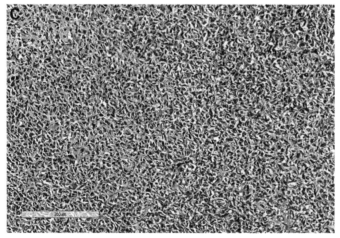

Fig. 5. (*A–J*). SEF of bone originally diagnosed as osteosarcoma with SEF-like appearance 17 years ago. (*A*) CT scan of left acetabular/pelvic lesion in 2005. (*B–F*) Histological features of the primary tumor showing (*B*) intra-osseous involvement by (*C*) sheets of angulated cells and

additional cases of SEF-like sarcomas with *YAP1::KMT2A* or reciprocal *KMT2A::YAP1* fusions have been described.[35,36,55] Although these sarcomas fit within the original morphologic description of SEF,[2] they lack immunohistochemical expression of MUC4 and canonical *EWSR/FUS* gene rearrangements typical of most SEF, suggesting they could represent a variant of MUC4-negative SEF.[36] Ultrastructural evidence of fibroblastic differentiation in *YAP1::KMT2A* sarcomas,[35] as well as the known heterogeneous expression of MUC4 in SEF,[18] would lend some support to this concept. However, limited gene expression data has shown that *KMT2A-*

Fig. 5. (*D*) only focal ribbon-like sclerosis simulating osteoid. The highly cellular areas merge with fibrotic zones (*E*). Higher magnification (*F*) shows a delicate lace-like deposition of matrix around individual cells. Innumerable and slowly progressive lung metastases

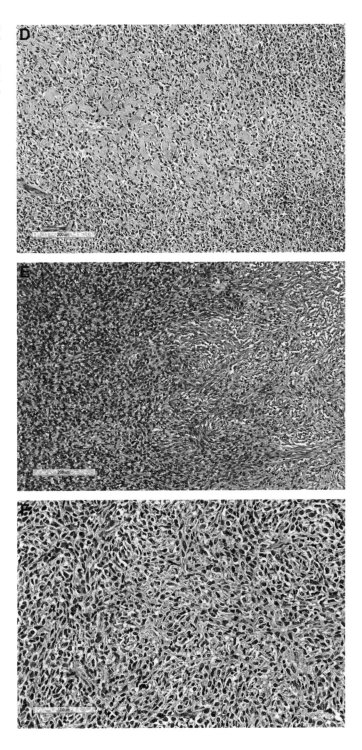

rearranged sarcomas cluster away from SEF and closer to myxofibrosarcoma, raising the possibility that they are a distinct entity separate from SEF.[34] Furthermore, sarcomas with *VIM::KMT2A* fusion are composed of cellular fascicles of uniform spindle cells with little morphologic resemblance to SEF,[56] and *KMT2A*-rearranged sarcomas with non-*YAP1* and non-*VIM* fusion partners also display a widely variant morphology.[35] Overall, these results underscore the importance of confirming the fusion partner in *KMT2A*-rearranged sarcomas, as the morphology and clinical

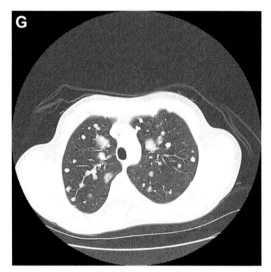

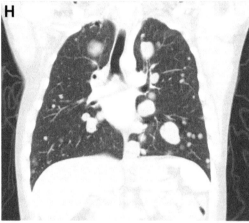

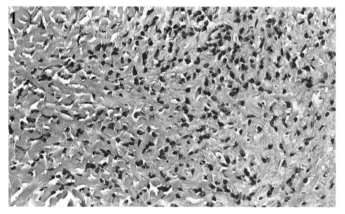

Fig. 5. (*G* and *H*) appeared 11 years after the primary tumor and continue to grow to date. Histologic sampling of lung metastases (*I* and

behavior may be very different. As such, only a subset of *YAP1::KMT2A* sarcomas may fall within the spectrum of SEF. Whether these sarcomas truly represent a distinct entity or a group of lesions with varying morphology and clinical behavior will continue to evolve with long-term follow-up and further molecular studies.

HISTOLOGICAL DIFFERENTIAL DIAGNOSIS

The differential diagnosis of SEF includes other tumors with epithelioid cells and dense fibrous matrix. Especially challenging is recognition on limited biopsy material since SEF can have a

Fig. 5. J) shows features like the original bone tumor, though blander. Note ropey collagen in (*I*). Molecular analysis of the lung metastasis revealed *EWSR1:: CREB3L2* fusion.

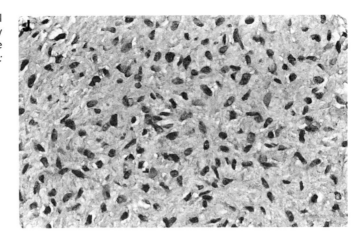

wide morphologic spectrum. Its propensity for bone involvement, occurrence as a primary bone tumor, and dense collagenous matrix simulating osteoid all cause confusion with osteosarcoma.[9] The latter typically shows, at least focally, unequivocal lace-like neoplastic bone formation around individual cells with extensive matrix calcification and pronounced nuclear atypia, along with strong diffuse nuclear positivity for SATB2.

Additionally, SEF can be mistaken for metastatic carcinoma due to its epithelioid morphology, particularly if it presents with synchronous bone metastases.[57] The closest morphologic mimickers include signet ring cell carcinoma and lobular breast carcinoma. SEF is typically negative for keratin, but many carcinomas can be positive for MUC4.[58,59] In addition to immunohistochemistry, correlation with clinical history and radiographic findings is helpful to distinguish SEF from metastatic carcinoma.

In soft tissue, the differential diagnosis also includes ossifying fibromyxoid tumor of soft parts (OFMT). OFMT is typically composed of small round epithelioid cells arranged in small nests, cords or trabeculae within a fibrous and myxoid stroma.[60] The nested cellular arrangements of OFMT occur in doublets and triplets in contrast to SEF, which has single cells or pseudo-alveoli. The nuclei of OFMT are usually rounded to spindled with smooth nuclear membranes, whereas SEF generally has more angulated nuclei. OFMT also tends to be more superficially located than SEF, occurring primarily in the subcutis. When present, the type of bone deposition seen in OFMT is quite distinctive as a peripheral rim in contrast to the metaplastic bone of SEF. Immunohistochemically, OFMT is positive for S100 protein in most cases and desmin in about 50%. Detection of

PHF1 gene rearrangements in some OFMT is another distinguishing feature.[61–63]

Rare cases of myoepithelial carcinoma may simulate SEF, with even focal expression of MUC4.[18] Unlike SEF, myoepithelial tumors also frequently show immunoreactivity for keratin, S100 protein, SOX10, SMA, and GFAP. Additionally, some myoepithelial tumors have *EWSR1* gene rearrangements; however, the fusion partners for *EWSR1* include *POU5F1* and *PBX1*,[64] rather than *CREB3L1* or *CREB3L2*.

SEF may also be confused with other tumors with sclerosing features, including sclerosing variants of rhabdomyosarcoma or lymphoma, although appropriate batteries of immunohistochemical stains will easily make the distinction. Hypercellular SEF composed of small cells closely resemble other small cell or round cell sarcomas, most notably Ewing sarcoma, poorly differentiated synovial sarcoma, cellular variants of extraskeletal myxoid chondrosarcoma, and mesenchymal chondrosarcoma.[9] NGS-fusion testing is critical in these cases. The gene fusions typically identified in SEF and tumors in the differential diagnosis are summarized in **Table 2**.

CLINICAL FEATURES OF SCLEROSING EPITHELIOID FIBROSARCOMA

AGE AND SEX DISTRIBUTION

In the largest published series to date, SEF showed a slight male predominance of 59% (30/51),[9] which is quite similar to that of LGFMS with 58% males (19/33).[40] The median age at first diagnosis was 45 years (range, 4 to 78 years), which is higher than typically seen in LGFMS showing a median age of 29 years (range, 6 to 52 years).[40]

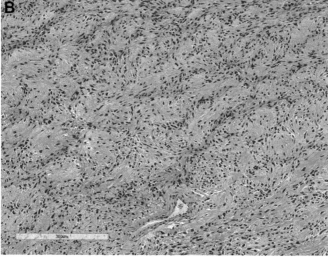

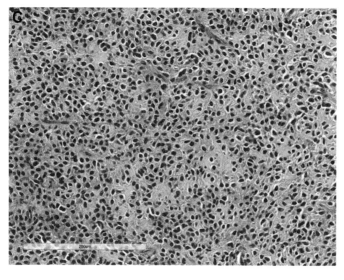

Fig. 6. (*A–C*). Recurrent low-grade fibro-myxoid sarcoma (LGFMS) of chest wall in another 53-year-old woman that showed focal dedifferentiation and *FUS::CREB3L2*. (*A*) Typical low-grade spindle cell areas with (*B*) "tigroid" areas and (*C*) small round cell foci of dedifferentiation that overlap with the appearance of SEF.

Fig. 7. (*A–E*). Recurrent LGFMS in the thigh with sclerosing features that arose after a 40-year hiatus. (*A*) Sclerotic, ropey matrix in local recurrence of thigh simulates SEF. (*B*) Hypocellular fibrous zone in local LGFMS recurrence. (*C–E*) Simultaneous intra-abdominal metastasis with (*C*) typical LGFMS areas as well as

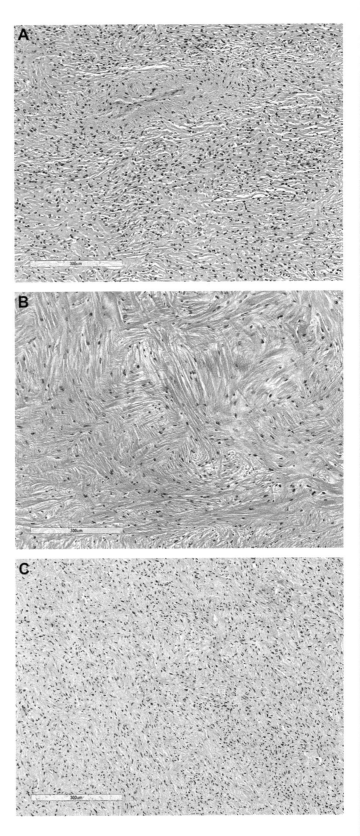

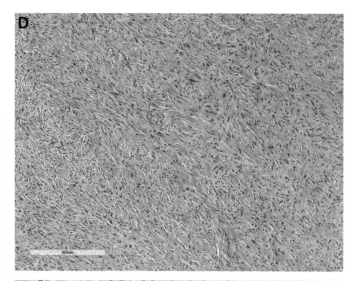

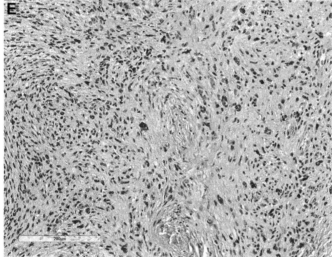

Fig. 7. (D) more collagenous, storiform zones and (E) multinucleated tumor cells in more cellular areas simulating dedifferentiated liposarcoma. Both the thigh recurrence and abdominal metastasis showed *FUS* rearrangement, and the abdominal metastasis was also negative for *MDM2* amplification by FISH.

While SEF commonly arises in middle-aged adults, rare cases have been reported in very young patients, including a 4-year-old male with a renal mass mimicking clear cell sarcoma of the kidney replete with synchronous bone metastases.[9] The typical clinical presentation of SEF is that of a slow growing (sometimes spanning decades) and painless mass.

PRIMARY AND METASTATIC TUMOR LOCATIONS

SEF has a wide anatomic distribution, having been described in many sites including the oral/maxillofacial region,[22,23] abdomen,[24] cecum,[25] distal pancreas,[26] kidney,[27] pelvis,[28] ovary,[29] and bone.[30,31,57] Among the most common primary

sites are the lower extremity, abdomen and visceral organs, limb girdle, trunk, and skeleton/bone. SEF has a propensity for deep soft tissue with deep fascial, periosteal, bone, and intra-cavity involvement. Periosteal involvement can lead to direct extension into bone with tumor morphologically resembling aponeuroses and suggesting a relationship with the Sharpey fiber-periosteal-endosteal system.[65] Multiple cases of SEF presenting with diffuse abdominal disease have been reported.[9,20] Extensive peritoneal sarcomatosis and visceral organ involvement is distinctly more common in SEF than LGFMS.

SEF metastasizes more quickly and extensively than LGFMS, most commonly to lung with other metastatic sites including bone, soft tissue, liver, brain, pleura, and lymph nodes, among others. It

Table 2
Fusion genes identified in SEF and tumors in differential diagnosis

Diagnosis	Most Common Fusion Genes	Less Common Fusion Genes
Sclerosing epithelioid fibrosarcoma	*EWSR1::CREB3L1*	*EWSR1::CREB3L2, FUS::CREB3L2, FUS::CREM, PAX5::CREB3L1, EWSR1::CREB3L3, YAP1::KMT2A HEY1::NCOA2, PRRX1::KMT2D*
Low-grade fibromyxoid sarcoma	*FUS::CREB3L2*	*FUS::CREB3L1, EWSR1::CREB3L1*
Ossifying fibromyxoid tumor	*EP400::PHF1*	*MEAF6::PHF1, EPC::PHF1, ZC3H7B::BCOR, CREBBEP::BCOR; KDM2A::WWTR1; PHF1::TFE3[67]*
Myoepithelial tumor	*EWSR1::POU5F1, EWSR1::PBX3, EWSR1::PBX1*	*EWSR1::ZNF44, EWSR1::KLF17, EWSR1::ATF11, EWSR1::VGLL1, FUS::KLF17, FUS::POU5F1[68–70]*
Ewing sarcoma	*EWSR1::FLI1, EWSR1::ERG*	*EWSR1:ETV1, EWSR1::ETV4, EWSR1::FEV, FUS::ERG, FUS::FEV, one member of FET family of genes and a member of ETS family of genes[71]*
Synovial sarcoma	*SS18::SSX1, SS18::SSX2*	*SS18::SSX4, SS18L1::SSX1[72,73]*
Extraskeletal myxoid chondrosarcoma	*EWSR1::NR4A3, TAF15::NR4A3*	*TCF12::NR4A3, TFG::NR4A3, FUS::NR4A3, HSPA8::NR4A3[74]*
Mesenchymal chondrosarcoma	*HEY1::NCOA2*	*IRF2BP2::CDX1[75,76]*

Fig. 8. Survival of SEF in comparison to survival of LGFMS from the same institution. SEF has a statistically significant poorer survival than LGFMS. (*From* Warmke LM, Meis JM. Sclerosing Epithelioid Fibrosarcoma: A Distinct Sarcoma with Aggressive Features. Am J Surg Pathol. 2021;45(3):317–328 reprinted with permission).

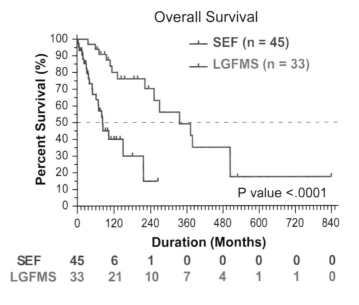

Table 3
SEF and LGFMS: Comparison of clinical features

	SEF (9)	LGFMS (40)
Age	45 years (4–78 years)	29 years (6–52 years)
Sex distribution	30 M: 21 F	19 M: 14 F
Tumor size	8.2 cm (3.2–29.0 cm)	9.4 cm (1.5–16.0 cm)
Tumor location	Wide anatomic distribution, propensity to involve intra-cavitary and periosteal sites	Wide anatomic distribution
Local recurrence rate	12/45 (27%)	21/33 (64%)
Metastatic rate	36/45 (80%)	15/33 (45%)
Metastatic sites	Lung most common, frequent bone and cranial involvement	Lung most common
Overall survival	Worse overall survival, metastasizes more quickly and extensively	Long, protracted clinical course

is far more likely to develop widespread osseous metastases (17/45, 38%) compared to LGFMS (2/33, 6%).[9]

IMAGING FINDINGS

SEF usually forms a well-demarcated mass, ranging in size from 3.2 to 29.0 cm with a median of 8.2 cm.[9] Findings on MR imaging may demonstrate a central area of low signal intensity on both T1-and T2-weighted images, surrounded by an area of intermediate signal intensity.[66] Heterogeneous enhancement on post-gadolinium images is frequently present. Primary SEF of bone often presents as a heterogeneous, osteolytic mass with bone destruction on CT. Areas showing calcification within the collagen can be misinterpreted as tumor osteoid.

TREATMENT

Early surgical intervention with R0 resection remains the most effective treatment for SEF. Re-excision is recommended for positive margins, and radiotherapy may be considered for optimal local disease control. Patients with unresectable disease may have palliative debulking with supportive end of life care. The effectiveness of systemic therapy is limited, as SEF is usually recalcitrant to most chemotherapy regimens. While only benefiting a minority of patients, partial response to doxorubicin/ifosfamide, as well as disease stabilization with doxorubicin monotherapy, has been reported.[37] Patients with widespread disease often progress despite chemotherapy and should be considered for participation in clinical trials. Although immune checkpoint blockade is ineffective in most

sarcomas, 2 patients with SEF, one with additional *PBRM1* mutation and one with a loss-of-function *JAK2* mutation, have shown clinical improvement and marked regression with ipilimumab and nivolumab therapy.[38] Given the high rate of local recurrence and metastasis, long-term clinical and radiologic follow-up is essential. Further investigation into novel therapeutic targets will hopefully provide more effective treatment in the future.

PROGNOSTIC FACTORS AND SURVIVAL

SEF has a much more aggressive clinical course than LGFMS with a local recurrence rate of 27-53%, metastatic rate of 43-80%, and overall mortality rate of 47%.[2,9] Primary tumor size, site, and patient sex have not been shown to correlate with outcome.[9]

With overall survival defined as the interval from histological diagnosis of SEF to death, the median overall survival in one series was 47.3 months (95% CI 25.0–131.9), and the metastasis-free survival in patients diagnosed with primary disease was 16.3 months (95% CI 5.3–20.6).[37] The overall survival of SEF is notably worse when compared to LGFMS (**Fig. 8**).[9] The clinical features of SEF in comparison to LGFMS are summarized in **Table 3**.

CLINICS CARE POINTS

- Any deep-seated soft tissue or bone mass could potentially be a SEF.
- Imaging features may be similar to a desmoid, high grade sarcoma or even an osteosarcoma.

- Histologic sampling with ancillary testing is necessary for accurate diagnosis.

- Wide surgical resection, if feasible, can prolong survival, although local recurrence, metastatic and mortality rates are high.

REFERENCES

1. Meis JM, Kindblom LG, Enzinger FM. Lab Invest 1994;70A.

2. Meis-Kindblom JM, Kindblom LG, Enzinger FM. Sclerosing epithelioid fibrosarcoma. A variant of fibrosarcoma simulating carcinoma. Am J Surg Pathol 1995;19(9):979–93.

3. Evans HL. Low-grade fibromyxoid sarcoma. A report of two metastasizing neoplasms having a deceptively benign appearance. Am J Clin Pathol 1987; 88(5):615–9.

4. Merck C, Angervall L, Kindblom LG, et al. Myxofibrosarcoma. A malignant soft tissue tumor of fibroblastic-histiocytic origin. A clinicopathologic and prognostic study of 110 cases using multivariate analysis. Acta Pathol Microbiol Immunol Scand Suppl 1983;282:1–40.

5. Kindblom LG, Merck C, Angervall L. The ultrastructure of myxofibrosarcoma. A study of 11 cases. Virchows Arch A Pathol Anat Histol 1979;381(2):121–39.

6. Erlandson RA, Woodruff JM. Role of electron microscopy in the evaluation of soft tissue neoplasms, with emphasis on spindle cell and pleomorphic tumors. Hum Pathol 1998;29(12):1372–81.

7. Reid R, Barrett A, Hamblen DL. Sclerosing epithelioid fibrosarcoma. Histopathology 1996;28(5):451–5.

8. Antonescu CR, Rosenblum MK, Pereira P, et al. Sclerosing epithelioid fibrosarcoma: a study of 16 cases and confirmation of a clinicopathologically distinct tumor. Am J Surg Pathol 2001;25(6):699–709.

9. Warmke LM, Meis JM. Sclerosing Epithelioid fibrosarcoma: a distinct sarcoma with aggressive features. Am J Surg Pathol 2021;45(3):317–28.

10. Peng Y, Chen T, Zhang D, et al. Primary sclerosing epithelioid fibrosarcoma of the kidney: a case report and review of the literature. Int J Surg Pathol 2022; 30(4):437–42.

11. Guillou L, Benhattar J, Gengler C, et al. Translocation-positive low-grade fibromyxoid sarcoma: clinicopathologic and molecular analysis of a series expanding the morphologic spectrum and suggesting potential relationship to sclerosing epithelioid fibrosarcoma: a study from the French Sarcoma Group. Am J Surg Pathol 2007;31(9):1387–402.

12. Rekhi B, Deshmukh M, Jambhekar NA. Low-grade fibromyxoid sarcoma: a clinicopathologic study of 18 cases, including histopathologic relationship with sclerosing epithelioid fibrosarcoma in a subset of cases. Ann Diagn Pathol 2011;15(5):303–11.

13. Rekhi B, Folpe AL, Deshmukh M, et al. Sclerosing epithelioid fibrosarcoma - a report of two cases with cytogenetic analysis of FUS gene rearrangement by FISH technique. Pathol Oncol Res 2011;17(1):145–8.

14. Storlazzi CT, Mertens F, Nascimento A, et al. Fusion of the FUS and BBF2H7 genes in low grade fibromyxoid sarcoma. Hum Mol Genet 2003;12(18): 2349–58.

15. Mertens F, Fletcher CD, Antonescu CR, et al. Clinicopathologic and molecular genetic characterization of low-grade fibromyxoid sarcoma, and cloning of a novel FUS/CREB3L1 fusion gene. Lab Invest 2005;85(3):408–15.

16. Prieto-Granada C, Zhang L, Chen HW, et al. A genetic dichotomy between pure sclerosing epithelioid fibrosarcoma (SEF) and hybrid SEF/low-grade fibromyxoid sarcoma: a pathologic and molecular study of 18 cases. Genes Chromosomes Cancer 2015;54(1):28–38.

17. Doyle LA, Moller E, Dal Cin P, et al. MUC4 is a highly sensitive and specific marker for low-grade fibromyxoid sarcoma. Am J Surg Pathol 2011;35(5):733–41.

18. Doyle LA, Wang WL, Dal Cin P, et al. MUC4 is a sensitive and extremely useful marker for sclerosing epithelioid fibrosarcoma: association with FUS gene rearrangement. Am J Surg Pathol 2012; 36(10):1444–51.

19. Wang WL, Evans HL, Meis JM, et al. FUS rearrangements are rare in 'pure' sclerosing epithelioid fibrosarcoma. Mod Pathol 2012;25(6):846–53.

20. Stockman DL, Ali SM, He J, et al. Sclerosing epithelioid fibrosarcoma presenting as intraabdominal sarcomatosis with a novel EWSR1-CREB3L1 gene fusion. Hum Pathol 2014;45(10):2173–8.

21. Arbajian E, Puls F, Magnusson L, et al. Recurrent EWSR1-CREB3L1 gene fusions in sclerosing epithelioid fibrosarcoma. Am J Surg Pathol 2014;38(6):801–8.

22. Elkins CT, Wakely PE Jr. Sclerosing epithelioid fibrosarcoma of the oral cavity. Head Neck Pathol 2011; 5(4):428–31.

23. Folk GS, Williams SB, Foss RB, et al. Oral and maxillofacial sclerosing epithelioid fibrosarcoma: report of five cases. Head Neck Pathol 2007;1(1):13–20.

24. Smith PJ, Almeida B, Krajacevic J, et al. Sclerosing epithelioid fibrosarcoma as a rare cause of ascites in a young man: a case report. J Med Case Rep 2008; 2:248.

25. Frattini JC, Sosa JA, Carmack S, et al. Sclerosing epithelioid fibrosarcoma of the cecum: a radiation-associated tumor in a previously unreported site. Arch Pathol Lab Med 2007;131(12):1825–8.

26. Bai S, Jhala N, Adsay NV, et al. Sclerosing epithelioid fibrosarcoma of the pancreas. Ann Diagn Pathol 2013;17(2):214–6.

27. Ertoy Baydar D, Kosemehmetoglu K, Aydin O, et al. Primary sclerosing epithelioid fibrosarcoma of kidney with variant histomorphologic features: report

of 2 cases and review of the literature. Diagn Pathol 2015;10:186.

28. Arya M, Garcia-Montes F, Patel HR, et al. A rare tumour in the pelvis presenting with lower urinary symptoms: 'sclerosing epithelioid fibrosarcoma'. Eur J Surg Oncol 2001;27(1):121–2.

29. Ogose A, Kawashima H, Umezu H, et al. Sclerosing epithelioid fibrosarcoma with der(10) t(10;17)(p11;q11). Cancer Genet Cytogenet 2004; 152(2):136–40.

30. Wojcik JB, Bellizzi AM, Dal Cin P, et al. Primary sclerosing epithelioid fibrosarcoma of bone: analysis of a series. Am J Surg Pathol 2014;38(11):1538–44.

31. Grunewald TG, von Luettichau I, Weirich G, et al. Sclerosing epithelioid fibrosarcoma of the bone: a case report of high resistance to chemotherapy and a survey of the literature. Sarcoma 2010;2010:431627.

32. Tsuda Y, Dickson BC, Dry SM, et al. Clinical and molecular characterization of primary sclerosing epithelioid fibrosarcoma of bone and review of the literature. Genes Chromosomes Cancer 2020; 59(4):217–24.

33. Righi A, Pacheco M, Pipola V, et al. Primary sclerosing epithelioid fibrosarcoma of the spine: a single-institution experience. Histopathology 2021; 78(7):976–86.

34. Puls F, Agaimy A, Flucke U, et al. Recurrent Fusions Between YAP1 and KMT2A in Morphologically Distinct Neoplasms Within the Spectrum of Low-grade Fibromyxoid Sarcoma and Sclerosing Epithelioid Fibrosarcoma. Am J Surg Pathol 2020;44(5):594–606.

35. Massoth LR, Hung YP, Nardi V, et al. Pan-sarcoma genomic analysis of KMT2A rearrangements reveals distinct subtypes defined by YAP1-KMT2A-YAP1 and VIM-KMT2A fusions. Mod Pathol 2020;33(11): 2307–17.

36. Kao YC, Lee JC, Zhang L, et al. Recurrent YAP1 and KMT2A gene rearrangements in a subset of MUC4-negative sclerosing epithelioid fibrosarcoma. Am J Surg Pathol 2020;44(3):368–77.

37. Chew W, Benson C, Thway K, et al. Clinical characteristics and efficacy of chemotherapy in sclerosing epithelioid fibrosarcoma. Med Oncol 2018;35(11): 138.

38. Doshi SD, Oza J, Remotti H, et al. Clinical benefit from immune checkpoint blockade in sclerosing epithelioid fibrosarcoma: a translocation-associated sarcoma. JCO Precis Oncol 2021;5:1–5.

39. Puls F, Magnusson L, Niblett A, et al. Non-fibrosing sclerosing epithelioid fibrosarcoma: an unusual variant. Histopathology 2016;68(5):760–3.

40. Evans HL. Low-grade fibromyxoid sarcoma: a clinicopathologic study of 33 cases with long-term follow-up. Am J Surg Pathol 2011;35(10):1450–62.

41. Forgo E, Hornick JL, Charville GW. MUC4 is expressed in alveolar rhabdomyosarcoma. Histopathology 2021;78(6):905–8.

42. Graham RP, Dry S, Li X, et al. Ossifying fibromyxoid tumor of soft parts: a clinicopathologic, proteomic, and genomic study. Am J Surg Pathol 2011;35(11): 1615–25.

43. Nagano N, Ishikawa N, Nagase M, et al. A case of cellular variants of Sclerosing epithelioid fibrosarcoma resembling Plasmacytoma/Myeloma: Diagnostic difficulty in the fine needle aspiration. Int J Surg Case Rep 2020;68:228–33.

44. Porteus C, Gan Q, Gong Y, et al. Sclerosing epithelioid fibrosarcoma: cytologic characterization with histologic, immunohistologic, molecular, and clinical correlation of 8 cases. J Am Soc Cytopathol 2020; 9(6):513–9.

45. Tsuchido K, Yamada M, Satou T, et al. Cytology of sclerosing epithelioid fibrosarcoma in pleural effusion. Diagn Cytopathol 2010;38(10):748–53.

46. Lau PP, Lui PC, Lau GT, et al. EWSR1-CREB3L1 gene fusion: a novel alternative molecular aberration of low-grade fibromyxoid sarcoma. Am J Surg Pathol 2013;37(5):734–8.

47. Arbajian E, Puls F, Antonescu CR, et al. In-depth genetic analysis of sclerosing epithelioid fibrosarcoma reveals recurrent genomic alterations and potential treatment targets. Clin Cancer Res 2017;23(23): 7426–34.

48. Dewaele B, Libbrecht L, Levy G, et al. A novel EWS-CREB3L3 gene fusion in a mesenteric sclerosing epithelioid fibrosarcoma. Genes Chromosomes Cancer 2017;56(9):695–9.

49. Murshed KA, Ammar A. Hybrid sclerosing epithelioid fibrosarcoma/low grade fibromyxoid sarcoma arising in the small intestine with distinct HEY1-NCOA2 gene fusion. Pathology 2020;52(5):607–10.

50. Folpe AL. 'I Can't Keep Up!': an update on advances in soft tissue pathology occurring after the publication of the 2020 World Health Organization classification of soft tissue and bone tumours. Histopathology 2022;80(1):54–75.

51. Meyer C, Burmeister T, Groger D, et al. The MLL recombinome of acute leukemias in 2017. Leukemia 2018;32(2):273–84.

52. Marx A, Belharazem D, Lee DH, et al. Molecular pathology of thymomas: implications for diagnosis and therapy. Virchows Arch 2021;478(1):101–10.

53. Santo EE, Ebus ME, Koster J, et al. Oncogenic activation of FOXR1 by 11q23 intrachromosomal deletion-fusions in neuroblastoma. Oncogene 2012;31(12):1571–81.

54. Watson S, Perrin V, Guillemot D, et al. Transcriptomic definition of molecular subgroups of small round cell sarcomas. J Pathol 2018;245(1):29–40.

55. Yoshida A, Arai Y, Tanzawa Y, et al. KMT2A (MLL) fusions in aggressive sarcomas in young adults. Histopathology 2019;75(4):508–16.

56. Almohsen SS, Griffin AM, Dickson BC, et al. VIM::KMT2A-rearranged sarcomas: a report of two

new cases confirming an entity with distinct histologic features. Genes Chromosomes Cancer 2023; 62(7):405–11.

57. Wang G, Eyden B. A primary sclerosing epithelioid fibrosarcoma of the pubic bone, with evidence of divergent epithelial differentiation. Ultrastruct Pathol 2010;34(2):99–104.

58. Andrianifahanana M, Moniaux N, Schmied BM, et al. Mucin (MUC) gene expression in human pancreatic adenocarcinoma and chronic pancreatitis: a potential role of MUC4 as a tumor marker of diagnostic significance. Clin Cancer Res 2001;7(12):4033–40.

59. Chauhan SC, Singh AP, Ruiz F, et al. Aberrant expression of MUC4 in ovarian carcinoma: diagnostic significance alone and in combination with MUC1 and MUC16 (CA125). Mod Pathol 2006; 19(10):1386–94.

60. Enzinger FM, Weiss SW, Liang CY. Ossifying fibromyxoid tumor of soft parts. A clinicopathological analysis of 59 cases. Am J Surg Pathol 1989; 13(10):817–27.

61. Folpe AL, Weiss SW. Ossifying fibromyxoid tumor of soft parts: a clinicopathologic study of 70 cases with emphasis on atypical and malignant variants. Am J Surg Pathol 2003;27(4):421–31.

62. Gebre-Medhin S, Nord KH, Moller E, et al. Recurrent rearrangement of the PHF1 gene in ossifying fibromyxoid tumors. Am J Pathol 2012;181(3):1069–77.

63. Graham RP, Weiss SW, Sukov WR, et al. PHF1 rearrangements in ossifying fibromyxoid tumors of soft parts: A fluorescence in situ hybridization study of 41 cases with emphasis on the malignant variant. Am J Surg Pathol 2013;37(11):1751–5.

64. Antonescu CR, Zhang L, Chang NE, et al. EWSR1-POU5F1 fusion in soft tissue myoepithelial tumors. A molecular analysis of sixty-six cases, including soft tissue, bone, and visceral lesions, showing common involvement of the EWSR1 gene. Genes Chromosomes Cancer 2010;49(12):1114–24.

65. Aaron JE. Periosteal Sharpey's fibers: a novel bone matrix regulatory system? Front Endocrinol 2012;3:98.

66. Christensen DR, Ramsamooj R, Gilbert TJ. Sclerosing epithelioid fibrosarcoma: short T2 on MR imaging. Skeletal Radiol 1997;26(10):619–21.

67. Carter CS, Patel RM. Ossifying fibromyxoid tumor: a review with emphasis on recent molecular advances and differential diagnosis. Arch Pathol Lab Med 2019;143(12):1504–12.

68. Flucke U, Mentzel T, Verdijk MA, et al. EWSR1-ATF1 chimeric transcript in a myoepithelial tumor of soft tissue: a case report. Hum Pathol 2012;43(5):764–8.

69. Komatsu M, Kawamoto T, Kanzawa M, et al. A novel EWSR1-VGLL1 gene fusion in a soft tissue malignant myoepithelial tumor. Genes Chromosomes Cancer 2020;59(4):249–54.

70. Suurmeijer AJH, Dickson BC, Swanson D, et al. A morphologic and molecular reappraisal of myoepithelial tumors of soft tissue, bone, and viscera with EWSR1 and FUS gene rearrangements. Genes Chromosomes Cancer 2020;59(6):348–56.

71. Kilpatrick SE, Reith JD, Rubin B. Ewing sarcoma and the history of similar and possibly related small round cell tumors: from whence have we come and where are we going? Adv Anat Pathol 2018; 25(5):314–26.

72. Sandberg AA, Bridge JA. Updates on the cytogenetics and molecular genetics of bone and soft tissue tumors. Synovial sarcoma. Cancer Genet Cytogenet 2002;133(1):1–23.

73. Storlazzi CT, Mertens F, Mandahl N, et al. A novel fusion gene, SS18L1/SSX1, in synovial sarcoma. Genes Chromosomes Cancer 2003;37(2): 195–200.

74. Urbini M, Astolfi A, Pantaleo MA, et al. HSPA8 as a novel fusion partner of NR4A3 in extraskeletal myxoid chondrosarcoma. Genes Chromosomes Cancer 2017;56(7):582–6.

75. Nyquist KB, Panagopoulos I, Thorsen J, et al. Whole-transcriptome sequencing identifies novel IRF2BP2-CDX1 fusion gene brought about by translocation t(1;5)(q42;q32) in mesenchymal chondrosarcoma. PLoS One 2012;7(11):e49705.

76. Wang L, Motoi T, Khanin R, et al. Identification of a novel, recurrent HEY1-NCOA2 fusion in mesenchymal chondrosarcoma based on a genome-wide screen of exon-level expression data. Genes Chromosomes Cancer 2012;51(2): 127–39.

CIC-Rearranged Sarcoma

Naohiro Makise, MD, PhD[a], Akihiko Yoshida, MD, PhD[b,c,*]

KEYWORDS

- *CIC* • *CIC*-rearranged sarcoma • *DUX4* • ETV4 • Ewing-like sarcoma • Fusion gene

---

Key points

- *CIC*-rearranged sarcoma is a distinct entity newly recognized by the fifth edition of the WHO classification.
- Histologic findings have been well characterized and are recognizable.
- Nuclear ETV4 and WT1 positivity are useful immunohistochemical findings.
- Molecular testing may fail to detect *CIC* fusion genes.
- *CIC*-rearranged sarcoma has a worse prognosis than Ewing sarcoma.

ABSTRACT

CIC-rearranged sarcoma is a rare type of small round cell sarcoma. The tumors often affect the deep soft tissues of patients in a wide age range. They are highly aggressive, respond poorly to chemotherapy, and have a worse outcome than Ewing sarcoma. *CIC*-rearranged sarcoma has characteristic and recognizable histology, including lobulated growth, focal myxoid changes, round to epithelioid cells, and minimal variation of nuclear size and shape. Nuclear ETV4 and WT1 expression are useful immunohistochemical findings. *CIC* fusion can be demonstrated using various methods; however, even next-generation sequencing suffers from imperfect sensitivity, especially for *CIC::DUX4*.

INTRODUCTION

Ewing sarcoma is a prototype of small round cell sarcoma and is currently defined as having gene fusions involving one member of the FET family of genes (usually *EWSR1*) and a member of the ETS family of transcription factors.[1] Recently, undifferentiated small round cell sarcomas without FET::ETS gene fusions have been recognized and referred to as "Ewing-like sarcoma." Subsequent advances in molecular pathology and phenotypic studies have established that "Ewing-like sarcoma" is not a single entity but encompasses several sarcoma types, distinct from Ewing sarcoma. The latest WHO classification recognizes 3 such tumor types: *CIC*-rearranged sarcoma, sarcoma with *BCOR* genetic alterations, and round cell sarcoma with *EWSR1*::non-ETS fusion.[1] *CIC*-rearranged sarcoma is the most common type, accounting for approximately 60% to 70% of cases of Ewing-like sarcoma.[2,3] Although the tumor is defined by *CIC* rearrangement, the classification is not solely based on the genotype because *CIC*-rearranged sarcomas exhibit characteristic histologic and immunohistochemical features on light microscopy. Furthermore, the molecular detection of *CIC* fusion is associated with inherent challenges, and evidence of gene fusion may not be always available in practice, even when using next-generation sequencing (NGS). According to the latest WHO classification of soft tissue and bone tumors, the detection of *CIC* fusion is not mandatory for diagnosis but is desirable in select cases.[1]

This review summarizes the contemporary knowledge regarding *CIC*-rearranged sarcomas

[a] Division of Surgical Pathology, Chiba Cancer Center, 666-2 Nitona-cho, Chuo-ku, Chiba-shi, Chiba, 260-8717, Japan; [b] Department of Diagnostic Pathology, National Cancer Center Hospital, Tokyo, Japan; [c] Rare Cancer Center, National Cancer Center, Tokyo, Japan
* Corresponding author. Department of Diagnostic Pathology, National Cancer Center Hospital, 5-1-1, Tsukiji, Chuo-ku, Tokyo 104-0045, Japan.
E-mail address: akyoshid@ncc.go.jp

Surgical Pathology 17 (2024) 141–151
https://doi.org/10.1016/j.path.2023.06.003
1875-9181/24/© 2023 Elsevier Inc. All rights reserved.

with an emphasis on the characteristic histologic and immunohistochemical features and diagnostic pitfalls, including false-negative results in molecular assays.

HISTORICAL PERSPECTIVE

CIC-rearranged sarcomas were likely submerged in the Ewing and other primitive sarcoma categories for a long time. Two articles published in 1992 described karyotypes t(4;19) (q35.1;q13.1) and t(4;19;12) (q35;q13.1;q13) in "embryonal rhabdomyosarcoma" and "undifferentiated/embryonal rhabdomyosarcoma," respectively.[4,5] A few subsequent reports of highly aggressive pediatric sarcomas with primitive round cell histology and focal myxoid features demonstrated t(4;19) (q35;q13.1).[6,7] However, it was not until in 2006 when Kawamura-Saito and colleadues[8] identified *CIC::DUX4* fusion transcripts in 2 "Ewing-like sarcomas" with t(4;19) (q35;q13) that the tumor became widely recognizable. Since then, more than 200 cases of *CIC*-rearranged sarcomas have been reported in the literature. Sugita and colleagues [9] described the first case of sarcoma with a variant *CIC* fusion, *CIC::FOXO4*. Sarcoma with *CIC::NUTM1* fusion is now established as a variant of *CIC*-rearranged sarcoma, rather than a *NUTM1*-rearranged neoplasm, based on overlapping phenotypes as well as transcriptomic and DNA methylation profiles with *CIC::DUX4* sarcomas.[10–12]

MOLECULAR PATHOGENESIS

CIC (19q13.2) encodes the transcriptional repressor CIC, which forms a complex with ATXN1 and ATXN1L.[13,14] CIC protein includes a high-mobility group (HMG) box DNA-binding domain, which recognizes T(G/C)AATG(A/G)A.[14] The *CIC* rearrangement consistently occurs intra-exonically, most often within exon 20, and rarely in exons 12, 15, 16, 18, or 19.[15] The base sequence at breakpoints often contains microhomology sequences and/or insertions.[15] In some cases, *CIC* is fused with untranslated regions of *DUX4* leading to a stop codon immediately after the breakpoint.[15,16] In the CIC fusion product, the C-terminal end of CIC is lost, whereas the HMG box DNA-binding domain is retained.[17] Consequently, the repressive function of CIC becomes converted to transactivating, and CIC target genes are aberrantly overexpressed, including the PEA3 family genes (*ETV1*, *ETV4*, and *ETV5*), *CCND2*, and *MUC5AC* among others.[8,18]

DUX4 is the most common *CIC* fusion partner (~95%). *DUX4* is located within the D4Z4 repeats of the subtelomeric regions in 4q35 and 10q26.

DUX4 plays an important role in early embryogenesis but is transcriptionally silenced in mature somatic tissues except in the testis and thymus.[19] *DUX4::IGH* fusion and subsequent DUX4 overexpression is a recurrent event in acute B-cell lymphoblastic leukemia in adolescents and young adults.[20] *CIC* fusion partners other than *DUX4* include *NUTM1* (15q14),[10,21–24] *NUTM2A* (10q23),[25,26] *LEUTX* (19q13),[27–29] *FOXO4* (Xq13),[9,30,31] *CREBBP* (16p13),[31] *AXL* (19q13),[29] *CITED1* (Xq13),[29] *SYT* (9q22),[29] and an unannotated region.[16] *CIC* fusion partner genes often contain transcriptional activating domains.

Other recurrent but inconsistent genetic aberrations include *MYC* amplification, trisomy 8,[32] and 1p loss.[33] The karyotypes are often simple, but sometimes more complex, particularly following chemotherapy.[34]

CLINICAL FEATURES

CIC-rearranged sarcomas can occur in patients of any age. However, they most commonly affect young adults with a median age of ~30 years. A slight male predilection is observed. The primary sites are deep soft tissues (~85%), including the extremities and body cavities. Superficial tumor locations, including the skin, have also been documented. Tumors uncommonly occur in the visceral organs (~10%). The affected viscera include the central nervous system (CNS), heart, lung, pleura, kidney, uterus, and gastrointestinal tract. Primary bone cases are rare (~5%) unlike Ewing sarcoma.[2,35] *CIC::NUTM1* sarcomas are predilected to the CNS and paravertebral regions with frequent bone involvement.[10,24] *CIC*-rearranged sarcomas are highly aggressive, often (~40%) associated with multiple metastases at diagnosis to sites including the lungs and lymph nodes.[36,37]

RADIOLOGIC FEATURES

On MRI, *CIC*-rearranged sarcoma is a deep, or sometimes superficial, large, lobulated mass (**Fig. 1**A). Characteristic findings include contrast enhancement, necrosis, perilesional edema, and flow voids.[37] Calcification is absent, and an average SUVmax was 13.2 based on one study.[37]

GROSS FEATURES

Macroscopically, *CIC*-rearranged sarcomas have a tan-white soft or fleshy appearance. They often show lobulated growth at the periphery accompanied by massive central necrosis and hemorrhage (**Fig. 1**B).

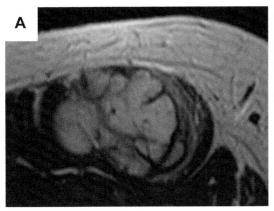
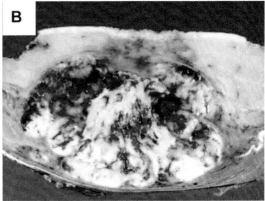

Fig. 1. Radiologic and gross findings of *CIC*-rearranged sarcoma. On MRI T2-weighted imaging, *CIC*-rearranged sarcoma presents as a large lobulated mass with heterogeneous signals (*A*). Grossly, *CIC*-rearranged sarcoma shows a tan-white fleshy appearance with lobulated growth, massive necrosis, and hemorrhage (*B*).

MICROSCOPIC FEATURES

At low magnification, the tumor periphery is often lobulated within a fibrotic background (**Figs. 2**A and B). Geographic necrosis and hemorrhage are common (see **Fig. 2**C). The neoplasm typically grows in diffuse sheets (see **Fig. 2**D). Focal myxoid changes with reticular or sieve-like patterns are common and diagnostically helpful (see **Fig. 2**E). The tumor may focally show a fascicular proliferation of spindle cells (see **Fig. 2**F). At higher magnification, the tumor consists of relatively uniform small round cells. However, careful inspection almost always reveals a mild degree of variation in the nuclear size and shape (ie, minimal nuclear pleomorphism, **Fig. 3**A). The nuclear chromatin is vesicular, and nucleoli are often readily visible. Epithelioid (see **Fig. 3**B) and rhabdoid (see **Fig. 3**C) cytomorphology may be focally observed. The cytoplasm is lightly eosinophilic with occasional clearing (see **Fig. 3**D). It is rare to observe an entirely uniform small round cell morphology that is indistinguishable from that of Ewing sarcoma (see **Fig. 3**E). Mitotic activity is brisk (see **Fig. 3**F). Rare morphologic variations include predominantly myxoid reticular growth and predominantly epithelioid cytomorphology. Cytoplasmic eosinophilic globules and cartilaginous differentiation are exceptional.[3] After neoadjuvant therapy, tumor cells may show marked pleomorphism.

IMMUNOHISTOCHEMICAL FEATURES

Most *CIC*-rearranged sarcomas are positive for CD99. However, the staining is often heterogeneous (**Fig. 4**A) unlike the diffuse strong membranous CD99 reactivity typically observed in Ewing sarcoma. ETV4 is the single most useful diagnostic marker with sensitivity and specificity of 90% to 95% among small round cell sarcomas.[15,38,39] (see **Fig. 4**B) Nuclear WT1 positivity, using a conventional N-terminus antibody, is another useful finding that is observed in 70% to 95% of cases (see **Fig. 4**C), which is often accompanied by cytoplasmic staining.[3,40] Other proposed positive markers include DUX4 (C-terminus).[41] *CIC::NUTM1* sarcoma shows diffuse nuclear expression of NUT protein (see **Fig. 4**D). The NUT staining pattern is not speckled unlike *BRD4/3::NUTM1* carcinoma.[10]

Similar to other fusion-driven sarcomas, *CIC*-rearranged sarcomas exhibit a "scrambled" immunophenotype that may lead to diagnostic challenges. Keratin (see **Fig. 4**E) and MUC4 can be focally positive.[3] TLE1 and calretinin are often expressed.[42] S100 protein, desmin, and synaptophysin labeling are rare. *CIC*-rearranged sarcomas commonly express ERG, and in a small subset of cases, CD31 is co-expressed usually with a heterogeneous staining pattern (see **Fig. 4**F).[43] NKX2.2, PAX7, BCOR, SOX10, myogenin, and CD45 are typically negative.[44]

DIAGNOSTIC MOLECULAR TESTS

FLUORESCENCE IN SITU HYBRIDIZATION (FISH)

CIC break-apart FISH is widely used because it requires only one unstained thin section and does not require the knowledge of partner genes. The positive break-apart pattern usually consists of split 5′ and 3′ signals in addition to normally fused 5′/3′ signals (**Fig. 5**A). In ∼10% of cases, isolated 5′ signals may be observed, which should not be dismissed as negative.[3,45] As with other FISH

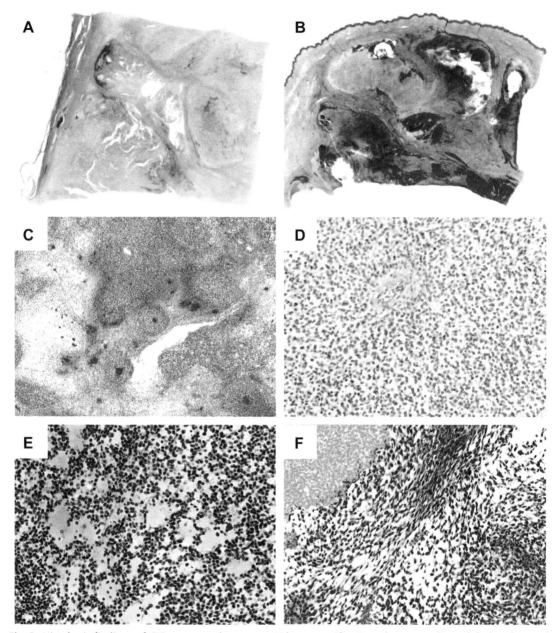

Fig. 2. Histologic findings of *CIC*-rearranged sarcoma. At low magnification, the tumor shows lobulated growth separated by fibrous septa (*A, B*). Geographic necrosis and hemorrhage are common (*C*). The round tumor cells grow in diffuse sheets (*D*). Focal myxoid change with a reticular growth pattern is characteristic and diagnostically helpful (*E*). Fascicular proliferation of tumor spindle cells may be focally observed (*F*).

assays, a quantitative assessment is the rule, and an optimal cutoff of the rearrangement-positive cell rate should be used (eg, 20%). Unfortunately, *CIC* break-apart FISH is not a highly sensitive method; 14% to 25% of cases produce negative signal patterns despite the presence of *CIC* fusions (see **Fig. 5**B).[15,16,44,45] Such false-negative FISH results are mostly associated with *CIC::-DUX4*. *CIC::LEUTX* may also be difficult to detect.

REVERSE TRANSCRIPTION POLYMERASE CHAIN REACTION (RT-PCR)

RT-PCR is also a widely used approach (see **Fig. 5**C).[2,34,42,46] However, owing to multiple intra-exonic breakpoints and non-*DUX4* fusion partners, the sensitivity of RT-PCR can be limited. In addition, fragmented RNA extracted from FFPE blocks can hamper reliable detection of fusion transcripts.

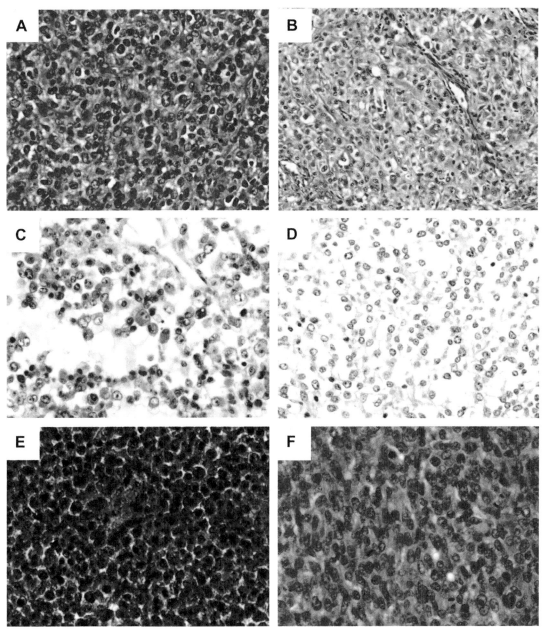

Fig. 3. Histologic findings of *CIC*-rearranged sarcoma. At high magnification, the round tumor cells have relatively uniform, but minimally pleomorphic, vesicular nuclei with distinct nucleoli and eosinophilic to amphophilic cytoplasm. The tumor may show round (*A*), epithelioid (*B*), and/or rhabdoid (*C*) cytomorphology. Cytoplasmic clearing is occasionally seen (*D*). The tumor rarely shows uniform small round cell morphology indistinguishable from Ewing sarcoma (*E*). Mitotic figures are numerous (*F*).

NEXT-GENERATION SEQUENCING

Targeted RNA sequencing and whole transcriptome sequencing are emerging diagnostic tools. Importantly, *CIC::DUX4* fusion is often missed when sequencing data are analyzed using fusion discovery algorithms, such as FusionMap, FusionFinder, ChimeraScan,[47] FusionSeq, STAR-Fusion,

Manta-Fusion, and TopHat-Fusion,[16] despite the chimeric reads being mapped onto the *CIC* gene. In such cases, *CIC::DUX4* fusions are not called in NGS reports but detected only after the characteristic tumor phenotype prompts a careful inspection of *CIC* reads on a genome viewer. The reason for these false-negative results is likely that the

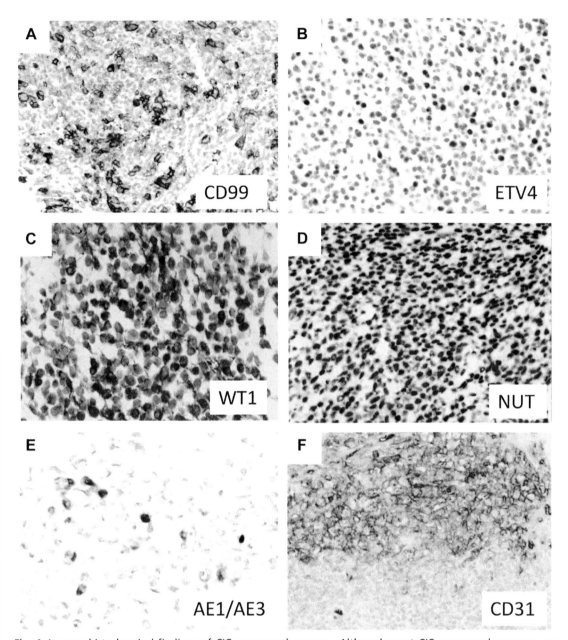

Fig. 4. Immunohistochemical findings of *CIC*-rearranged sarcoma. Although most *CIC*-rearranged sarcomas are positive for CD99, the staining is often focal and heterogeneous (*A*). ETV4 is a highly sensitive and specific marker (*B*). Nuclear WT1 positivity, often accompanied by cytoplasmic staining, is relatively sensitive and specific to *CIC*-rearranged sarcomas (*C*). *CIC::NUTM1*-positive examples show diffuse nuclear NUT expression (*D*). Keratin can be focally positive (*E*). CD31 (*F*) and ERG may be co-expressed in a heterogeneous manner.

chimeric reads are filtered out as noise because of the repetitive nature of *DUX4* sequences. In contrast, *CIC::LEUTX*,[27,28] *CIC::FOXO4*,[9,30] and *CIC::NUTM1*[10,21–24] are often detected using fusion discovery algorithms. Several methods, such as ArcherDX FusionPlex, have reportedly detected *CIC::DUX4* fusion transcripts.[25,48–50]

DIFFERENTIAL DIAGNOSIS

Compared with *Ewing sarcoma*, lobulation, focal myxoid change, focal spindle cell change, and prominent nucleoli are significantly more common in *CIC*-rearranged sarcomas.[3] The tumor cells, which have more pleomorphic nuclei and ampler cytoplasm, are more cohesive than those of Ewing

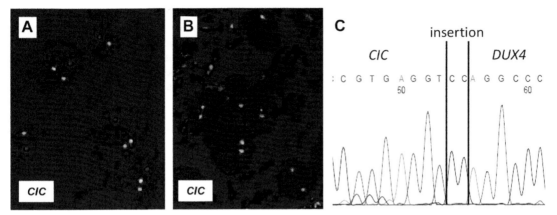

Fig. 5. Molecular testing for *CIC*-rearranged sarcoma. *CIC* break-apart FISH usually shows split signals in *CIC::-DUX4* sarcomas (*A*, split green and orange signals indicate *CIC* rearrangements). However, approximately 15% of *CIC::DUX4* sarcomas show negative FISH results (*B*). In this particular case (shown in B), RT-PCR successfully detected a *CIC::DUX4* fusion transcript (*C*).

sarcoma. Ewing sarcoma is typically positive for CD99 in a diffuse strong membranous pattern, unlike the heterogeneous staining in *CIC*-rearranged sarcomas. More specific Ewing markers NKX2.2 and PAX7 are usually negative in *CIC*-rearranged sarcoma, and conversely, Ewing sarcoma is negative for nuclear WT1 and ETV4.[44] The genetic hallmark of Ewing sarcoma is the fusion between *EWSR1/FUS* and ETS family genes, such as *FLI1* and *ERG*.

Sarcomas with *BCOR* genetic alterations typically present as a uniform oval-to-spindle cell proliferation within a variably myxoid or vascular stroma. The tumor is often positive for BCOR and SATB2, but negative for ETV4 and WT1.[44]

Desmoplastic small round cell tumor (DSRCT) shows nests of round cells in a desmoplastic stroma and may mimic *CIC*-rearranged sarcoma. DSRCT is characterized by the expression of keratin and desmin. Although nuclear WT1 (C-terminus) is expressed in DSRCT, nuclear WT1 (N-terminus) expression is lacking. DSRCT is driven by *EWSR1::WT1* fusion.

CIC-rearranged sarcoma can be misdiagnosed as cellular *extraskeletal myxoid chondrosarcoma (EMC)* when myxoid changes predominate with a reticular growth pattern. EMC typically presents in middle-aged to older patients, and the diagnosis of EMC is worth revisiting in children and young adults, particularly when the tumor is aggressive. EMC is negative for ETV4 and WT1 but is variably positive for S100 protein and neuroendocrine markers. EMC harbors *NR4A3* fusions.

Predominantly epithelioid morphology in *CIC*-rearranged sarcomas may cause misinterpretation as carcinoma or mesothelioma, especially in biopsies from the body cavities. *CIC*-rearranged

sarcomas can be positive for keratin, and they often express WT1 and calretinin, and sometimes D2-40; such a "mesothelioma panel" should be cautiously used when diagnosing round cell malignancies.[3] BAP1 loss and HEG1 expression are useful findings for mesothelioma, and claudin-4 is sensitive for carcinoma.

Co-expression of ERG and CD31 in a small subset of *CIC*-rearranged sarcoma may be a source of confusion with *epithelioid angiosarcoma*, which is further confounded by occasional hemorrhagic cleft-like spaces and intracytoplasmic vacuolation in *CIC*-rearranged sarcomas.[43] *CIC*-rearranged sarcomas lack true vascular structures. ERG and CD31 expression in *CIC*-rearranged sarcoma are heterogeneous, often focal and weak, rather than uniformly diffuse and strong as observed in angiosarcoma.

Other considerations include *rhabdomyosarcoma* and switch/sucrose non-fermentable (SWI/SNF)-deficient tumors, including *epithelioid sarcoma*. *CIC*-rearranged sarcomas consistently lack myogenin and myoD1 labeling and always retain SMARCB1/INI1 and SMARCA4/BRG1 expression.

TREATMENT AND PROGNOSIS

An optimal treatment strategy is yet to be established. However, patients often receive multimodal treatments, including surgery, chemotherapy, and/or radiation. Patients in advanced stages tend to be treated with Ewing-based chemotherapy; however, the response is often poor, with rare exceptions.[31,51] The treatment effect reportedly did not differ significantly between regimens oriented to Ewing sarcoma and those for high-grade spindle cell sarcoma.[51] Notably, however, there have been a few prolonged survivors who were treated with Ewing-type regimens.[51] The response to pazopanib, pembrolizumab, and paclitaxel was reportedly also poor.[31,43]

The 5 year overall survival rate is 17% to 43%,[3,31,35] and median survival is 12 to 18 months.[3,31,51] The prognosis of these patients is significantly worse than that of patients with Ewing sarcoma.[3,35] No prognostic factors have been identified.

AREAS OF FUTURE INVESTIGATION

ATXN1/ATXN1L-REARRANGED SARCOMAS

In recent years, a small number of sarcomas have been reported in the CNS that exhibit overlapping phenotypes or DNA methylation profiles with *CIC*-rearranged sarcomas in the absence of *CIC* fusions. Although a few of them contained frame-shift mutations in the *CIC* gene,[12,52] the majority of these tumors harbored alternative fusions involving *ATXN1* or *ATXN1L*, including *ATXN1/ATXIN1L::NUTM2A*,[53] *ATXN1::DUX4*,[52,54] and *ATXN1::NUTM1*.[55] ATXN1 and its paralog ATXN1L form a transcriptional suppressor complex with CIC through their evolutionary conserved AXH domain and play an important role in normal brain development.[56] ATXN1/ATXN1L::-NUTM1/NUTM2A/DUX4 fusion proteins retain the complex-forming AXH domain of ATXN1/ATXN1L.[13] These tumors appear to activate CIC target genes in a manner similar to that in *CIC*-rearranged sarcomas. Based on their overlapping histology, immunophenotype, and/or DNA methylation profile, *ATXN1/ATXN1L*-rearranged sarcomas likely belong to the family of *CIC*-rearranged sarcomas, suggesting an expansion of the disease concept.[54]

QUEST FOR NOVEL THERAPEUTIC OPTIONS

CIC-rearranged sarcomas respond poorly to existing chemotherapy regimens and novel therapeutic strategies are urgently required. Potentially effective treatments that have been investigated in preclinical studies include bortezomib (a 26S proteasome inhibitor), crizotinib (a multitargeted tyrosine kinase inhibitor),[57] dinaciclib (CDK2 inhibitor),[58] linsitinib (IGF-1R inhibitor),[59] BCI (DUSP6 inhibitor),[60] iP300w (P300/CBP inhibitor),[61] adavosertib (WEE1 inhibitor),[62] and dactolisib (dual AKT/mTOR inhibitor) with trabectedin.[63]

SUMMARY

CIC-rearranged sarcomas are relatively common among the tumors previously known as Ewing-like sarcomas. The tumors have characteristic and recognizable histology and immunoprofile, and such phenotypic findings often help in diagnosis. Molecular detection of *CIC* fusions, even using next-generation sequencing, may provide false-negative results, highlighting the critical value of careful phenotypic studies. *CIC*-rearranged sarcoma is highly aggressive and the prognosis is significantly worse than that of Ewing sarcoma.

CLINICS CARE POINTS

- *CIC*-rearranged sarcoma is a newly established type of small round cell sarcoma.
- Histologic findings have been well characterized and are recognizable.
- Nuclear ETV4 and WT1 positivity are useful immunohistochemical findings.
- Molecular testing may fail to detect *CIC* fusion genes.
- *CIC*-rearranged sarcoma is more aggressive than Ewing sarcoma.

FUNDING/CONFLICT OF INTEREST

This work was supported in part by JSPS, Japan KAKENHI (Grant Numbers JP20K16167 and JP21K06919) and the Rare Cancer Grant of National Cancer Center Hospital (G007). A. Yoshida reports grants from Daiichi Sankyo and personal fees from Eisai outside the submitted work. N. Makise has nothing to disclose.

ACKNOWLEDGMENTS

The authors acknowledge Hajime Kageyama and Hiroshi Kato for their excellent technical assistance.

REFERENCES

1. WHO Classification of Tumours Editorial Board. In: WHO classification of tumours soft tissue and bone tumours. 5th edition. Lyon: IARC; 2020.
2. Italiano A, Sung YS, Zhang L, et al. High prevalence of CIC fusion with double-homeobox (DUX4) transcription factors in EWSR1-negative undifferentiated small blue round cell sarcomas. Genes Chromosomes Cancer 2012;51(3):207–18.
3. Yoshida A, Goto K, Kodaira M, et al. CIC-rearranged Sarcomas: A Study of 20 Cases and Comparisons

With Ewing Sarcomas. Am J Surg Pathol 2016;40(3): 313–23.

4. Urumov IJ, Manolova Y. Cytogenetic analysis of an embryonal rhabdomyosarcoma cell line. Cancer Genet Cytogenet 1992;61(2):214–5.

5. Roberts P, Browne CF, Lewis IJ, et al. 12q13 abnormality in rhabdomyosarcoma. A nonrandom occurrence? Cancer Genet Cytogenet 1992;60(2):135–40.

6. Richkind KE, Romansky SG, Finklestein JZ. t(4;19)(q35;q13.1): a recurrent change in primitive mesenchymal tumors? Cancer Genet Cytogenet 1996;87(1):71–4.

7. Somers GR, Shago M, Zielenska M, et al. Primary subcutaneous primitive neuroectodermal tumor with aggressive behavior and an unusual karyotype: case report. Pediatr Dev Pathol 2004;7(5):538–45.

8. Kawamura-Saito M, Yamazaki Y, Kaneko K, et al. Fusion between CIC and DUX4 up-regulates PEA3 family genes in Ewing-like sarcomas with t(4;19)(q35;q13) translocation. Hum Mol Genet 2006;15(13):2125–37.

9. Sugita S, Arai Y, Tonooka A, et al. A novel CIC-FOXO4 gene fusion in undifferentiated small round cell sarcoma: a genetically distinct variant of Ewing-like sarcoma. Am J Surg Pathol 2014;38(11): 1571–6.

10. Le Loarer F, Pissaloux D, Watson S, et al. Clinicopathologic Features of CIC-NUTM1 Sarcomas, a New Molecular Variant of the Family of CIC-Fused Sarcomas. Am J Surg Pathol 2019;43(2):268–76.

11. Watson S, Perrin V, Guillemot D, et al. Transcriptomic definition of molecular subgroups of small round cell sarcomas. J Pathol 2018;245(1):29–40.

12. Sturm D, Orr BA, Toprak UH, et al. New Brain Tumor Entities Emerge from Molecular Classification of CNS-PNETs. Cell 2016;164(5):1060–72.

13. Lam YC, Bowman AB, Jafar-Nejad P, et al. ATAXIN-1 interacts with the repressor Capicua in its native complex to cause SCA1 neuropathology. Cell 2006;127(7):1335–47.

14. Tanaka M, Yoshimoto T, Nakamura T. A double-edged sword: The world according to Capicua in cancer. Cancer Sci 2017;108(12):2319–25.

15. Yoshida A, Arai Y, Kobayashi E, et al. CIC break-apart fluorescence in-situ hybridization misses a subset of CIC-DUX4 sarcomas: a clinicopathological and molecular study. Histopathology 2017;71(3):461–9.

16. Kao YC, Sung YS, Chen CL, et al. ETV transcriptional upregulation is more reliable than RNA sequencing algorithms and FISH in diagnosing round cell sarcomas with CIC gene rearrangements. Genes Chromosomes Cancer 2017;56(6):501–10.

17. Fores M, Simon-Carrasco L, Ajuria L, et al. A new mode of DNA binding distinguishes Capicua from other HMG-box factors and explains its mutation patterns in cancer. PLoS Genet 2017;13(3): e1006622.

18. Yoshimoto T, Tanaka M, Homme M, et al. CIC-DUX4 Induces Small Round Cell Sarcomas Distinct from Ewing Sarcoma. Cancer Res 2017;77(11): 2927–37.

19. Mocciaro E, Runfola V, Ghezzi P, et al. DUX4 Role in Normal Physiology and in FSHD Muscular Dystrophy. Cells 2021;10(12).

20. Yasuda T, Tsuzuki S, Kawazu M, et al. Recurrent DUX4 fusions in B cell acute lymphoblastic leukemia of adolescents and young adults. Nat Genet 2016; 48(5):569–74.

21. Biederman LE, Lee K, Yeager ND, et al. CIC::NUTM1 sarcoma mimicking primitive myxoid mesenchymal tumour of infancy: report of a case. Histopathology 2022;81(1):131–3.

22. Mangray S, Kelly DR, LeGuellec S, et al. Clinicopathologic Features of a Series of Primary Renal CIC-rearranged Sarcomas With Comprehensive Molecular Analysis. Am J Surg Pathol 2018;42(10): 1360–9.

23. Schaefer IM, Dal Cin P, Landry LM, et al. CIC-NUTM1 fusion: A case which expands the spectrum of NUT-rearranged epithelioid malignancies. Genes Chromosomes Cancer 2018;57(9):446–51.

24. Yang S, Liu L, Yan Y, et al. CIC-NUTM1 Sarcomas Affecting the Spine. Arch Pathol Lab Med 2022; 146(6):735–41.

25. Mantilla JG, Ricciotti RW, Chen E, et al. Detecting disease-defining gene fusions in unclassified round cell sarcomas using anchored multiplex PCR/targeted RNA next-generation sequencing-Molecular and clinicopathological characterization of 16 cases. Genes Chromosomes Cancer 2019;58(10): 713–22.

26. Sugita S, Arai Y, Aoyama T, et al. NUTM2A-CIC fusion small round cell sarcoma: a genetically distinct variant of CIC-rearranged sarcoma. Hum Pathol 2017;65:225–30.

27. Huang SC, Zhang L, Sung YS, et al. Recurrent CIC Gene Abnormalities in Angiosarcomas: A Molecular Study of 120 Cases With Concurrent Investigation of PLCG1, KDR, MYC, and FLT4 Gene Alterations. Am J Surg Pathol 2016;40(5):645–55.

28. Song K, Huang Y, Xia CD, et al. A case of CIC-rearranged sarcoma with CIC-LEUTX gene fusion in spinal cord. Neuropathology 2022;42(6):555–62.

29. Linos K, Dermawan JK, Bale T, et al. Expanding the Molecular Diversity of CIC-Rearranged Sarcomas With Novel and Very Rare Partners. Mod Pathol 2023;36(5):100103.

30. Solomon DA, Brohl AS, Khan J, et al. Clinicopathologic features of a second patient with Ewing-like sarcoma harboring CIC-FOXO4 gene fusion. Am J Surg Pathol 2014;38(12):1724–5.

31. Connolly EA, Bhadri VA, Wake J, et al. Systemic treatments and outcomes in CIC-rearranged Sarcoma: A national multi-centre clinicopathological

series and literature review. Cancer Med 2022;11(8): 1805–16.

32. Smith SC, Buehler D, Choi EY, et al. CIC-DUX sarcomas demonstrate frequent MYC amplification and ETS-family transcription factor expression. Mod Pathol 2015;28(1):57–68.

33. Lazo de la Vega L, Hovelson DH, Cani AK, et al. Targeted next-generation sequencing of CIC-DUX4 soft tissue sarcomas demonstrates low mutational burden and recurrent chromosome 1p loss. Hum Pathol 2016;58:161–70.

34. Choi EY, Thomas DG, McHugh JB, et al. Undifferentiated small round cell sarcoma with t(4;19)(q35;q13.1) CIC-DUX4 fusion: a novel highly aggressive soft tissue tumor with distinctive histopathology. Am J Surg Pathol 2013;37(9):1379–86.

35. Antonescu CR, Owosho AA, Zhang L, et al. Sarcomas With CIC-rearrangements Are a Distinct Pathologic Entity With Aggressive Outcome: A Clinicopathologic and Molecular Study of 115 Cases. Am J Surg Pathol 2017;41(7):941–9.

36. Machado I, Cruz J, Lavernia J, et al. Superficial EWSR1-negative undifferentiated small round cell sarcoma with CIC/DUX4 gene fusion: a new variant of Ewing-like tumors with locoregional lymph node metastasis. Virchows Arch 2013;463(6):837–42.

37. Brady EJ, Hameed M, Tap WD, et al. Imaging features and clinical course of undifferentiated round cell sarcomas with CIC-DUX4 and BCOR-CCNB3 translocations. Skeletal Radiol 2021; 50(3):521–9.

38. Hung YP, Fletcher CD, Hornick JL. Evaluation of ETV4 and WT1 expression in CIC-rearranged sarcomas and histologic mimics. Mod Pathol 2016; 29(11):1324–34.

39. Le Guellec S, Velasco V, Perot G, et al. ETV4 is a useful marker for the diagnosis of CIC-rearranged undifferentiated round-cell sarcomas: a study of 127 cases including mimicking lesions. Mod Pathol 2016;29(12):1523–31.

40. Specht K, Sung YS, Zhang L, et al. Distinct transcriptional signature and immunoprofile of CIC-DUX4 fusion-positive round cell tumors compared to EWSR1-rearranged Ewing sarcomas: further evidence toward distinct pathologic entities. Genes Chromosomes Cancer 2014;53(7):622–33.

41. Siegele B, Roberts J, Black JO, et al. DUX4 Immunohistochemistry Is a Highly Sensitive and Specific Marker for CIC-DUX4 Fusion-positive Round Cell Tumor. Am J Surg Pathol 2017;41(3):423–9.

42. Yamada Y, Kuda M, Kohashi K, et al. Histological and immunohistochemical characteristics of undifferentiated small round cell sarcomas associated with CIC-DUX4 and BCOR-CCNB3 fusion genes. Virchows Arch 2017;470(4):373–80.

43. Kojima N, Arai Y, Satomi K, et al. Co-expression of ERG and CD31 in a subset of CIC-rearranged

sarcoma: a potential diagnostic pitfall. Mod Pathol 2022;35(10):1439–48.

44. Yoshida A. Ewing and Ewing-like sarcomas: A morphological guide through genetically-defined entities. Pathol Int 2022;73(1):12–26.

45. Cocchi S, Gamberi G, Magagnoli G, et al. CIC rearranged sarcomas: A single institution experience of the potential pitfalls in interpreting CIC FISH results. Pathol Res Pract 2022;231:153773.

46. Gambarotti M, Benini S, Gamberi G, et al. CIC-DUX4 fusion-positive round-cell sarcomas of soft tissue and bone: a single-institution morphological and molecular analysis of seven cases. Histopathology 2016;69(4):624–34.

47. Panagopoulos I, Gorunova L, Bjerkehagen B, et al. The "grep" command but not FusionMap, FusionFinder or ChimeraScan captures the CIC-DUX4 fusion gene from whole transcriptome sequencing data on a small round cell tumor with t(4;19)(q35;q13). PLoS One 2014;9(6):e99439.

48. Loke BN, Lee VKM, Sudhanshi J, et al. Novel exon-exon breakpoint in CIC-DUX4 fusion sarcoma identified by anchored multiplex PCR (Archer FusionPlex Sarcoma Panel). J Clin Pathol 2017;70(8):697–701.

49. Brcic I, Brodowicz T, Cerroni L, et al. Undifferentiated round cell sarcomas with CIC-DUX4 gene fusion: expanding the clinical spectrum. Pathology 2020;52(2):236–42.

50. Ko JS, Marusic Z, Azzato EM, et al. Superficial sarcomas with CIC rearrangement are aggressive neoplasms: A series of eight cases. J Cutan Pathol 2020;47(6):509–16.

51. Brahmi M, Gaspar N, Gantzer J, et al. Patterns of care and outcome of CIC-rearranged sarcoma patients: A nationwide study of the French sarcoma group. Cancer Med 2023;12(7):7801–7.

52. Pratt D, Kumar-Sinha C, Cieslik M, et al. A novel ATXN1-DUX4 fusion expands the spectrum of 'CIC-rearranged sarcoma' of the CNS to include non-CIC alterations. Acta Neuropathol 2021;141(4): 619–22.

53. Xu F, Viaene AN, Ruiz J, et al. Novel ATXN1/ATXN1L::NUTM2A fusions identified in aggressive infant sarcomas with gene expression and methylation patterns similar to CIC-rearranged sarcoma. Acta Neuropathol Commun 2022;10(1):102.

54. Satomi K, Ohno M, Kubo T, et al. Central nervous system sarcoma with ATXN1::DUX4 fusion expands the concept of CIC-rearranged sarcoma. Genes Chromosomes Cancer 2022;61(11):683–8.

55. Siegfried A, Masliah-Planchon J, Roux FE, et al. Brain tumor with an ATXN1-NUTM1 fusion gene expands the histologic spectrum of NUTM1-rearranged neoplasia. Acta Neuropathol Commun 2019;7(1):220.

56. Lu HC, Tan Q, Rousseaux MW, et al. Disruption of the ATXN1-CIC complex causes a spectrum of

neurobehavioral phenotypes in mice and humans. Nat Genet 2017;49(4):527–36.

57. Oyama R, Takahashi M, Yoshida A, et al. Generation of novel patient-derived CIC- DUX4 sarcoma xenografts and cell lines. Sci Rep 2017;7(1):4712.

58. Okimoto RA, Wu W, Nanjo S, et al. CIC-DUX4 oncoprotein drives sarcoma metastasis and tumorigenesis via distinct regulatory programs. J Clin Invest 2019;129(8):3401–6.

59. Nakai S, Yamada S, Outani H, et al. Establishment of a novel human CIC-DUX(4) sarcoma cell line, Kitra-SRS, with autocrine IGF-1R activation and metastatic potential to the lungs. Sci Rep 2019;9(1):15812.

60. Lin YK, Wu W, Ponce RK, et al. Negative MAPK-ERK regulation sustains CIC-DUX4 oncoprotein expression in undifferentiated sarcoma. Proc Natl Acad Sci U S A 2020;117(34):20776–84.

61. Bosnakovski D, Ener ET, Cooper MS, et al. Inactivation of the CIC-DUX4 oncogene through P300/CBP inhibition, a therapeutic approach for CIC-DUX4 sarcoma. Oncogenesis 2021;10(10):68.

62. Ponce RKM, Thomas NJ, Bui NQ, et al. WEE1 kinase is a therapeutic vulnerability in CIC-DUX4 undifferentiated sarcoma. JCI Insight 2022;7(6).

63. Carrabotta M, Laginestra MA, Durante G, et al. Integrated Molecular Characterization of Patient-Derived Models Reveals Therapeutic Strategies for Treating CIC-DUX4 Sarcoma. Cancer Res 2022;82(4):708–20.

Pleomorphic Dermal Sarcoma

Jasmine S. Saleh, MD, MPH[a,b], Carli P. Whittington, MD[a,b], Scott C. Bresler, MD, PhD[a,b], Rajiv M. Patel, MD[a,b,c],*

KEYWORDS

- Pleomorphic dermal sarcoma • Atypical fibroxanthoma • Malignant fibrous histiocytoma
- Undifferentiated pleomorphic sarcoma • Sarcoma

Key points

- Pleomorphic dermal sarcoma is a rare cutaneous neoplasm of purported mesenchymal differentiation that exists along a clinicopathologic spectrum with atypical fibroxanthoma.

- Compared to atypical fibroxanthoma, pleomorphic dermal sarcoma demonstrates deeper dermal and/or subcutaneous involvement as well as more aggressive histopathological features.

- Pleomorphic dermal sarcoma is considered a diagnosis of exclusion and requires an appropriate immunohistochemical work-up to exclude other spindle cell neoplasms, including melanoma, squamous cell carcinoma, leiomyosarcoma, and angiosarcoma.

- Pleomorphic dermal sarcoma exhibits low-grade malignant behavior with a modest rate of local recurrence and distant metastasis.

- Wide local surgical excision is the first-line treatment for pleomorphic dermal sarcoma.

ABSTRACT

Pleomorphic dermal sarcoma (PDS) is a rare cutaneous/subcutaneous neoplasm of purported mesenchymal differentiation that exists along a clinicopathologic spectrum with atypical fibroxanthoma (AFX). While PDS and AFX share histopathologic and immunohistochemical features, PDS exhibits deeper tissue invasion and has a higher rate of metastasis and local recurrence than AFX. Given its aggressive clinical course, early recognition and clinical management of PDS are essential for optimizing patient outcomes. This review aims to provide a brief overview of the clinicopathologic and molecular features, prognosis, and treatment of PDS.

INTRODUCTION

Pleomorphic dermal sarcoma (PDS) refers to a dermal-based tumor that shares clinical, morphologic, and immunohistochemical characteristics with atypical fibroxanthoma (AFX).[1–4] PDS demonstrates more aggressive histopathological features, including invasion of deep dermal and/or subcutaneous tissue, tumor necrosis, lymphovascular invasion, and/or perineural infiltration.[1,3,4] Distinguishing PDS from AFX is critical, as they differ in their propensity to invade, locally recur, and metastasize.[1,4,5] While AFX is confined to the dermis and is associated with an overall favorable prognosis, PDS is aggressive, more invasive, and tends to be infiltrative with a significantly higher rate of metastasis and local recurrence.[1,4]

HISTORY

Pleomorphic dermal sarcoma was previously categorized as a so-called "malignant fibrous histiocytoma" (MFH).[6–9] Subsequently, as many tumors regarded as MFH were able to be more precisely classified into distinct pathologic

[a] Department of Pathology, University of Michigan, 2800 Plymouth Road, Building 35, Ann Arbor, MI 48109, USA; [b] Department of Dermatology, University of Michigan, 1500 E. Medical Center Drive, Ann Arbor, MI 48109, USA; [c] Cutaneous Pathology, WCP Laboratories, Inc., Maryland Heights, MO, USA
* Corresponding author.
E-mail address: rajivpat@med.umich.edu

Surgical Pathology 17 (2024) 153–158
https://doi.org/10.1016/j.path.2023.06.007
1875-9181/24/© 2023 Elsevier Inc. All rights reserved.

entities, many with specific lines of differentiation, unclassifiable sarcomas were re-designated as *undifferentiated pleomorphic sarcomas*.[8,10,11] However, it has been recognized that undifferentiated pleomorphic sarcomas involving deep soft tissue have a higher metastatic rate than superficially occurring tumors.[5,8,11] Hence, in light of this marked difference in biologic behavior, the term *pleomorphic dermal sarcoma* was proposed to refer specifically to cutaneous neoplasms involving the dermis and subcutaneous tissue.[6–8]

CLINICAL FEATURES

PDS typically develops on chronically sun-damaged skin, particularly the scalp of elderly patients, with a male predilection (M:F = 7:1)[1,12] Clinically, PDS presents as a rapidly growing, often ulcerated, nodular or polypoid lesion that may measure up to 6 cm in diameter.[1,12–14] Compared to AFX, PDS is usually larger, more asymmetric, and less well-circumscribed.[1] Ulceration, crusting, and/or bleeding are seen in most cases of PDS.[12]

MICROSCOPIC FEATURES

PDS is a large, asymmetric, and poorly circumscribed tumor with a diffusely infiltrative or pushing growth pattern into the subcutaneous tissue (**Fig. 1**).[10,12,15,16] Similar to AFX, which lacks broad infiltration into the underlying subcutis (**Fig. 2**), PDS is composed of highly atypical pleomorphic spindled and epithelioid cells with admixed multinucleated giant cells.[5,11,14,16] The neoplastic cells demonstrate abundant, and occasionally vacuolated, cytoplasm and hyperchromatic or vesicular nuclei with multiple nucleoli.[3,13,16,17] Numerous atypical mitoses are frequently present.[12] Ulceration, tumor necrosis, perineural invasion, and/or lymphovascular invasion may be seen.[12,14,16,17]

While the histopathologic features of classic PDS are well-recognized, various histologic variants have been reported in the literature. PDS may reveal prominent myxoid stroma, which may lead to confusion with myxofibrosarcoma.[12,14,18] Desmoplastic stroma may be seen and can resemble desmoplastic melanoma or squamous cell carcinoma.[12,14] PDS may demonstrate pseudoangiomatous changes, which are characterized by intratumoral blood-filled spaces, hemorrhage, and intracytoplasmic vacuoles.[1,12] Rarely, PDS may show a storiform growth pattern, keloidal stromal change, and/or admixed osteoclast-like giant cells.[1,12,14,16,19]

IMMUNOHISTOCHEMISTRY

PDS is considered a diagnosis of exclusion and requires an appropriate immunohistochemical work-up to exclude the possibility of other malignant spindle cell neoplasms, including melanoma, sarcomatoid squamous cell carcinoma, leiomyosarcoma, and angiosarcoma.[2,4,18,20] Although AFX/PDS shows positivity for CD10 in 95% to 100% of cases, the marker is nonspecific with limited or no diagnostic utility. Therefore, in the setting of CD10 negativity, a diagnosis of AFX/PDS cannot be entirely ruled out. Vimentin similarly has no diagnostic value other than perhaps to demonstrate general intact immunoreactivity of the tissue. Cytokeratins (CKs), particularly high molecular weight CKs such as CK5/6 and CK903 (34bE12), may aid in distinguishing PDS from poorly differentiated/sarcomatoid squamous cell carcinoma.[14,18] Of note, p63 expression has been rarely observed in PDS.[12,14,18] Lack of S100 and SOX10 expression may help exclude a diagnosis of desmoplastic or spindle cell melanoma; however, it is important to note that PDS may show intratumoral S100-positive dendritic cells.[14,18,20,21] Furthermore, multinucleated giant cells in PDS may also stain positively for Melan-A/Mart-1.[12,14,17,18,22] Melan-A/MART-1 expression in PDS is thought to be due to the cross-reactivity with an unidentified antigen or staining against fragments of melanocytic antigens.[14,22]

Although up to 70% of PDS cases express smooth muscle actin (SMA), typically in a "tram-track-like" pattern indicative of myofibroblastic differentiation, the neoplastic cells are negative for desmin, which can help exclude leiomyosarcoma.[12,18,21] PDS can express CD31 and FLI1, which can be a diagnostic pitfall for cutaneous angiosarcoma.[12,18] However, it is consistently negative for CD34 and ERG.[12,18]

Benign simulants of PDS include symplastic trichodiscoma and spindle cell/pleomorphic lipoma.[23] Trichodiscomas typically include intimately associated hyperplastic folliculosebaceous epithelium, while spindle cell/pleomorphic lipoma consistently expresses CD34 with nuclear loss of Rb expression. Additionally, brisk mitotic activity is not characteristic of either entity. Rarely, atypical dermatofibromas may be mistaken for PDS despite their rarity of presentation in the head and neck area. Microscopic evaluation of atypical dermatofibroma will reveal vague circumscription at low power with collagen entrapment at the periphery as well as epidermal hyperplasia overlying the lesion.

MOLECULAR PATHOLOGY FEATURES

AFX and PDS have been shown to harbor UV-signature mutations, particularly involving

Fig. *1.* Pleomorphic dermal sarcoma (PDS). Scanning magnification demonstrates a poorly circumscribed, highly cellular tumor (*A*) with focal invasion into subcutaneous tissue (*B*). Higher magnification shows atypical epithelioid to focally spindled cells with ample cytoplasm, variable nucleoli, and nuclear pleomorphism. Multinucleated giant cells and numerous mitotic figures are identified (*C*).

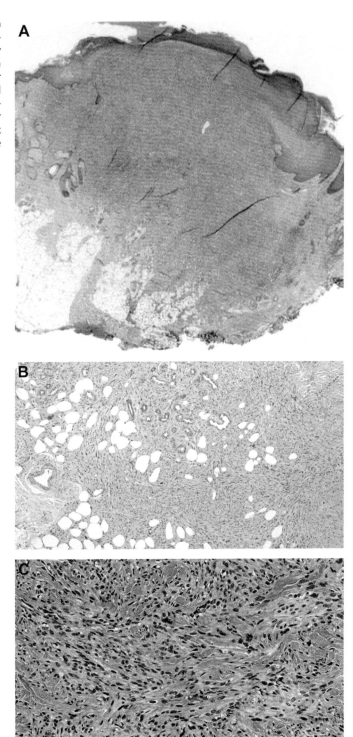

TP53 and *TERT*.[1,12,17,21,24] *TERT* promoter mutations, which are thought to allow cells to proliferate continuously without entering apoptosis or senescence, are the most frequent mutation in these entities.[17,21,24] In a recent study, *TERT* promoter mutations were found in 76% of PDS cases and 93% of AFX cases.[24] In addition, AFX and PDS share multiple genetic alterations,

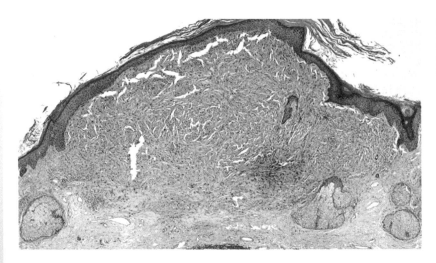

Fig. 2. Atypical fibroxanthoma (AFX). Scanning magnification shows a nodular tumor within the dermis.

including *FAT1, NOTCH1/2, CDKN2A, COL1A1,* and *PDGFR,* suggesting that they represent a spectrum of genetically related tumors.[1,4,5,15]

While AFX and PDS share molecular features, recent studies have identified activating RAS mutations in PDS, but not in AFX.[20,25] This implies that this gene mutation may be unique to the development of PDS.

DIFFERENTIAL DIAGNOSIS

PDS may mimic sarcomatoid squamous cell carcinoma, malignant melanoma, leiomyosarcoma, and/or angiosarcoma. The patient's clinical presentation, as well as histologic features and immunohistochemical markers, may aid in the differential diagnosis (**Table 1**).[1,12,18,20]

PROGNOSIS

PDS exhibits low-grade malignant behavior with a local recurrence risk of 20% to 35% and a metastatic risk of 10% to 20%.[1,5,10,12,15,26] In contrast, AFX has a local recurrence rate of 4.6% to 11.3% and a metastatic potential of 1% to 2%.[10,15,17,27] Complete surgical excision is the primary treatment modality.[3,28] Radiation therapy and/or chemotherapy may provide additional benefits for unresectable, locally recurrent, or regionally metastatic disease.[16,29,30] Routine follow-up with close clinical surveillance is recommended

Table 1
Differential diagnosis of pleomorphic dermal sarcoma

	Clinical Presentation	Microscopic Features	Immunohistochemistry
Sarcomatoid squamous cell carcinoma	Similar to PDS	Epidermal connection Squamous differentiation	Cytokeratin p63
Melanoma	+/− pigmentation	Overlying junctional involvement/ melanoma in situ	SOX10 S100
Leiomyosarcoma	Trunk and extremities	Spindle cells with elongated, blunt-ended, or cigar-shaped nuclei Cells show eosinophilic-staining cytoplasm and perinuclear vacuoles	SMA Desmin h-caldesmon
Angiosarcoma	+/− bluish to erythematous discoloration	Anastomosing vascular spaces	CD34 ERG

in patients diagnosed with PDS because of the potential risk for local recurrence and metastasis.[16,30]

SUMMARY

AFX and PDS tumors share many clinicopathologic, immunohistochemical, and genetic features. Compared to AFX, PDS shows more aggressive histologic features, including invasion of deep dermal and/or subcutaneous tissue, tumor necrosis, lymphovascular invasion, and/or perineural infiltration. PDS may mimic other spindle cell neoplasms and requires an appropriate immunohistochemical work-up to exclude these possibilities. Given the risk of local recurrence and distant metastasis, early recognition and management of PDS is critical for optimizing patient outcomes.

CLINICS CARE POINTS

- PDS is a rare cutaneous/subcutaneous neoplasm that predominantly arises on chronically sun-damaged skin of the elderly, particularly the scalp. There is a male predominance.

- It is important to differentiate PDS from its more benign-behaving counterpart, AFX, because of its risk for metastasis.

- The patient's clinical presentation, histologic features, and immunohistochemical profile may aid in distinguishing PDS from other spindle cell neoplasms, including melanoma, squamous cell carcinoma, leiomyosarcoma, and angiosarcoma, among others.

- Complete and wide surgical excision is the primary treatment modality for PDS.

DISCLOSURE

The authors have nothing to disclose.

REFERENCES

1. Brenn T. Soft Tissue Special Issue: Cutaneous Pleomorphic Spindle Cell Tumors. Head Neck Pathol 2020;14(1):109–20.
2. Cesinaro AM, Gallo G, Tramontozzi S, et al. Atypical fibroxanthoma and pleomorphic dermal sarcoma: A reappraisal. J Cutan Pathol 2021;48(2):207–10.
3. Kim JI, Choi YJ, Seo HM, et al. Case of Pleomorphic Dermal Sarcoma of the Eyelid Treated with Micrographic Surgery and Secondary Intention Healing. Ann Dermatol 2016;28(5):632–6.
4. Ørholt M, Abebe K, Aaberg F, et al. Immunohistochemical Characteristics of Atypical Fibroxanthoma and Pleomorphic Dermal Sarcoma: A Systematic Review and Meta-Analysis. Am J Dermatopathol 2022;44(12):913–20.
5. Bowe CM, Godhania B, Whittaker M, et al. Pleomorphic dermal sarcoma: a clinical and histological review of 49 cases. Br J Oral Maxillofac Surg 2021;59(4):460–5.
6. McCalmont TH. Correction and clarification regarding AFX and pleomorphic dermal sarcoma. J Cutan Pathol 2012;39(1):8.
7. McCalmont TH. AFX: what we now know. J Cutan Pathol 2011;38(11):853–6.
8. Cohen PR. Cutaneous undifferentiated pleomorphic sarcoma is a pleomorphic dermal sarcoma. Dermatol Online J 2020;26(5):13030.
9. Tillman BN, Liu JC. Cutaneous Sarcomas. Otolaryngol Clin North Am 2021;54(2):369–78.
10. Cohen AJ, Talasila S, Lazarevic B, et al. Pleomorphic dermal sarcoma of the scalp: Review of management and distinguishing features from atypical fibroxanthoma. JAAD Case Rep 2022;29:123–6.
11. Piras V, Ferreli C, Atzori L, et al. Atypical fibroxanthoma/pleomorphic dermal sarcoma of the scalp with aberrant expression of HMB-45: a pitfall in dermatopathology. Pathologica 2020;112(2):105–9.
12. Brenn T. Pleomorphic dermal neoplasms: a review. Adv Anat Pathol 2014;21(2):108–30.
13. Aigner B, Ugurel S, Kaddu S, et al. Cutaneous sarcomas: update on selected fibrohistiocytic and myofibroblastic tumors. Hautarzt 2014;65(7):614–22.
14. Miller K, Goodlad JR, Brenn T. Pleomorphic dermal sarcoma: adverse histologic features predict aggressive behavior and allow distinction from atypical fibroxanthoma. Am J Surg Pathol 2012;36(9):1317–26.
15. Logan IT, Vroobel KM, le Grange F, et al. Pleomorphic dermal sarcoma: Clinicopathological features and outcomes from a 5-year tertiary referral centre experience. Cancer Rep 2022;5(11):e1583.
16. Soleymani T, Tyler Hollmig S. Conception and Management of a Poorly Understood Spectrum of Dermatologic Neoplasms: Atypical Fibroxanthoma, Pleomorphic Dermal Sarcoma, and Undifferentiated Pleomorphic Sarcoma. Curr Treat Options Oncol 2017;8(8):50.
17. Hussein MR. Atypical fibroxanthoma: new insights. Expert Rev Anticancer Ther 2014;14(9):1075–88.
18. Tardío JC, Pinedo F, Aramburu JA, et al. Pleomorphic dermal sarcoma: a more aggressive neoplasm than previously estimated. J Cutan Pathol 2016;43(2):101–12.
19. Ardakani NM, Pearce R, Wood BA. Pleomorphic dermal sarcoma with osteosarcoma-like and chondrosarcoma-like elements. Pathology 2016;48(1):86–9.

20. López L, Vélez R. Atypical Fibroxanthoma. Arch Pathol Lab Med 2016;40(4):376–9.

21. Costigan DC, Doyle LA. Advances in the clinico-pathological and molecular classification of cutaneous mesenchymal neoplasms. Histopathology 2016;68(6):776–95.

22. Helbig D, Mauch C, Buettner R, et al. Immunohisto-chemical expression of melanocytic and myofibro-blastic markers and their molecular correlation in atypical fibroxanthomas and pleomorphic dermal sarcomas. J Cutan Pathol 2018;45(12):880–5.

23. Aghighi M, Andea AA, Patel RM, et al. Spindle Cell/ Pleomorphic Lipoma With Trichodiscoma-like Epithelial Hyperplasia Mimicking Atypical Fibroxan-thoma/Pleomorphic Dermal Sarcoma. Am J Derma-topathol 2022;44(10):764–7.

24. Griewank KG, Schilling B, Murali R, et al. TERT pro-moter mutations are frequent in atypical fibroxantho-mas and pleomorphic dermal sarcomas. Mod Pathol 2014;27(4):502–8.

25. Helbig D, Quaas A, Mauch C, et al. Copy number variations in atypical fibroxanthomas and pleomor-phic dermal sarcomas. Oncotarget 2017;8(65): 109457–67.

26. Lo ACQ, McDonald S, Wong KY. Case of pleomor-phic dermal sarcoma with systematic review of dis-ease characteristics, outcomes and management. BMJ Case Rep 2021;14(8):e244522.

27. Sharma SR, Meligonis G. and Todd P. Uncommon skin cancer: pleomorphic dermal sarcoma, *BMJ Case Rep*, 2018, 2018, bcr-2018-224483.

28. Lonie S, Yau B, Henderson M, et al. Management of pleomorphic dermal sarcoma. ANZ J Surg 2020; 90(11):2322–4.

29. Jang N, Shin HW, Yoon KC. Locally Advanced Pleo-morphic Dermal Sarcoma of the Forearm. J Hand Surg Am 2021;46(6):521.

30. Messina V, Cope B, Keung EZ, et al. Management of Skin Sarcomas. Surg Oncol Clin N Am 2022;31(3): 511–25.

Printed and bound by CPI Group (UK) Ltd, Croydon, CR0 4YY

03/10/2024

01040363-0014